Temple Street Children's Hospital

Temple Street Children's Hospital

An Illustrated History

BARRY KENNERK

NEW ISLAND

Temple Street Children's Hospital: An Illustrated History

First published in 2014
by New Island Books,
16 Priory Hall Office Park,
Stillorgan,
County Dublin,
Republic of Ireland.

www.newisland.ie

PRINT ISBN: 978-1-84840-389-5
EPUB ISBN: 978-1-84840-390-1
MOBI ISBN: 978-1-84840-391-8

British Library Cataloguing Data.
A CIP catalogue record for this book is available from the British Library.

Typeset by JVR Creative, India
Cover design by Mariel Deegan and New Island
Printed by ScandBook AB, Sweden

10 9 8 7 6 5 4 3 2 1

Contents

Acknowledgements

I would like to begin by thanking the team at New Island for taking on this project as well as author Cecelia Ahern, whose foreword has captured the essence of what Temple Street means to the children and families it serves. Thereafter, I would like to acknowledge my friends and colleagues for their support and enthusiasm. They include our photographer, Tommy Nolan, Thomas Prior, Yvonne Thompson, the projects team and all my colleagues in the neurosurgical department. Where possible, I have tried to expand upon our knowledge, but recognition is also due to past hospital historians, Dr F.O.C. Meenan and Sr Magdalene McPartlan, RSC, who saw to it that new staff members understood their roles in furthering the mission first undertaken by the Sisters of Charity founder, Mother Mary Aikenhead. I reserve special thanks to Joe Duffy and the team at RTE's *Liveline*, the *Evening Herald*, *Ireland's Own* and to Pat O'Rourke at *The People Group*. Each of these publications helped to spread the word about the project in its early stages and, as a result, many people (some of whom would have been difficult to locate otherwise) came forward to contribute their photographs and memories. The National Photographic Archive and Irish Architectural Archive also assisted in locating old plans and photographs of the hospital – some of which appear here.

Throughout its long history, Temple Street Children's Hospital has been about ordinary men and women doing extraordinary things on behalf of the children of Ireland. It is both an honour and a privilege to write about them and their achievements.

Ar dheis Dé go raibh a n-anama.

A Note on Sources

I n preparing this book for publication, I have visited several archives, each of which is abbreviated below. In addition, I have drawn heavily on the hospital's own papers, none of which have been catalogued at the time of writing. Perhaps this book may serve as the inspiration to preserve this material for future generations.

Dublin Diocesan Archives	DDA
Irish Architectural Archive	IAA
Irish Military Archives	IMA
National Archives of Ireland	NAI
National Library of Ireland	NLI
Registry of Deeds	ROD
Royal College of Physicians in Ireland	RCPI
Sisters of Charity Archive	SCA
Temple Street Hospital Archive	TSA
University College Dublin Archive	UCDA

A Note on Terminology

The Sisters of Charity is underpinned by the rule of St. Ignatius, founder of the Jesuit order. The priests had a 'father rector' in each community. Likewise, the sisters answered to a 'mother rectress'. Today, the latter term has become somewhat archaic and from the early twentieth century onwards, the head of the congregation at Temple Street was increasingly referred to as 'mother superioress' or 'mother superior' – the title which is used throughout this book.

*Dedicated to Professor Ian Temperley in grateful
appreciation for everything I hold most dear*

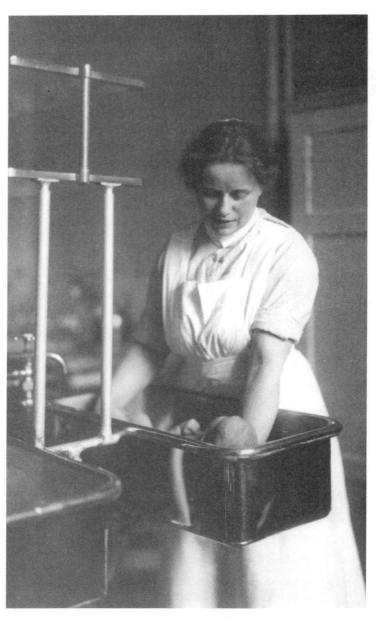

A nurse washes a baby with care at Temple Street Hospital, c.1930,
(Hospital collection)

Foreword by Cecelia Ahern

The very same day that I was asked to contribute to this book, I was trying to figure out what to write when my then three-year-old daughter, who seemed a little down, shared with me her recent lesson that her heroes, *superheroes*, aren't real after all. They are just cartoons, or movies. Not living in this world. She was crushed by the idea. I told her that she was wrong; that of course superheroes exist.

> '*They wear costumes?*'
> '*Of course they do.*'
> '*They fight the bad guys?*'
> '*Absolutely.*'

Fire-fighters, police, paramedics, doctors, nurses all put their costumes on and help save the lives of people every single day. Sometimes we might walk past them and not even know that we have been in the company of somebody who has managed the incredible feat of saving another person's life, or who has nursed a person back to health. They look like ordinary people, though they do extraordinary things, and they themselves might not even realise how extraordinary they are, because as a mother it is not just the obvious things that can help – it is the smallest things, such as a caring word, a supportive phrase, a comforting smile, which can help heal the worries of a parent when their child is sick.

My connections with Temple Street go back far. My mother worked in the kitchens at the age of fourteen on her summer holidays and it is where my parents' families have dashed in the moments we all dread. I have spent time in Temple Street with a child of mine, I have slept on that floor beside that cot, listening to the sounds of machines, seeing tubes going from an instrument into my child and wondering and fearing about everything a parent worries about in a moment like that. The angels in Temple Street have kept us going. Their everyday has been to care, to help, to heal, to comfort. We bring our babies into this world and we rely so much on those in the wards to help keep them there.

Temple Street Hospital has existed at this address since 1879. From then to now there are catalogues of evidence of the wonderful, beautiful, magical, heart-lifting and heart-breaking stories of those who passed through its halls and inhabited its rooms; stories which have remained silent for so many years.

You know the expression, if those walls could talk....Well, now they are talking, on the pages of this book.

Introduction

Temple Street Children's Hospital is now a household name in Ireland. At the time of writing, it stands as the only remaining children's institution in the heart of Dublin City. It was founded just twenty years after Great Ormond Street Hospital in London and continues to maintain a proud tradition in caring for sick children from all over the country.

Like many of my colleagues, I first came to know the hospital as a patient. I have a vivid memory of being rushed there as a toddler in the late 1970s, when I put my hand on a burning log in my granny's fireplace. The visit left a blurred impression of hard tiles, nurses and lights. Later, in the mid 1990s, I started my first summer job as a kitchen porter, swabbing down the terracotta-tiled floors. Since then, I have filled many other roles on either a casual or full-time basis. I remember the meningitis scare during the mid-1990s, when I could hardly leave the desk in A&E and the street was crammed with travelling people's vans. Equally, I have witnessed the strength of that same community fill the chapel as they prayed for the recovery of a sick child – the most powerful affirmation of faith imaginable.

As father to two girls, I have also seen the hospital from a parent's perspective – an anxious drive to A&E in the early hours; sweating in a lead apron while a fractured arm or chest is being X-rayed, the worry while waiting for test results to come through.

Life at Temple Street is multi-faceted – too varied perhaps for a complete history to be written and this book makes no such pretence. Every day, the building plays mute witness to the miraculous and the tragic. Its doors are kept open by a diverse team that includes not just doctors and nurses, but maintenance personnel, household staff, porters and allied health professionals. Indeed, the biggest challenge in writing this book has not simply been drawing together their stories into a single narrative, but also situating each account in its historical context. As a result, some departments will not feature or may receive only scant mention but that bears no reflection on the value of their work.

Over the past two years, I have interviewed over sixty past staff and patients, some of whom have since passed away. For many of them, recounting their time at Temple Street was clearly a cathartic experience. This is their book, and I hope that it does them justice.

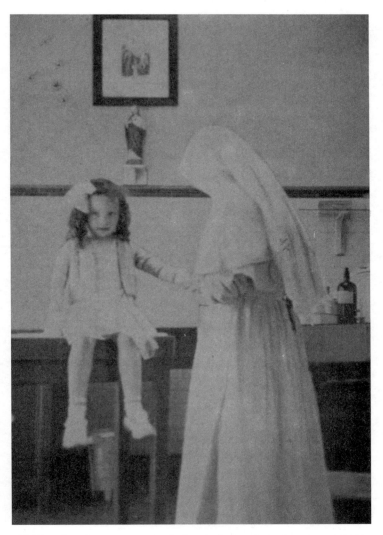

Child undergoing treatment in the hospital outpatients department, 1914.
Note the Sacred Heart statue in the background. (Hospital collection)

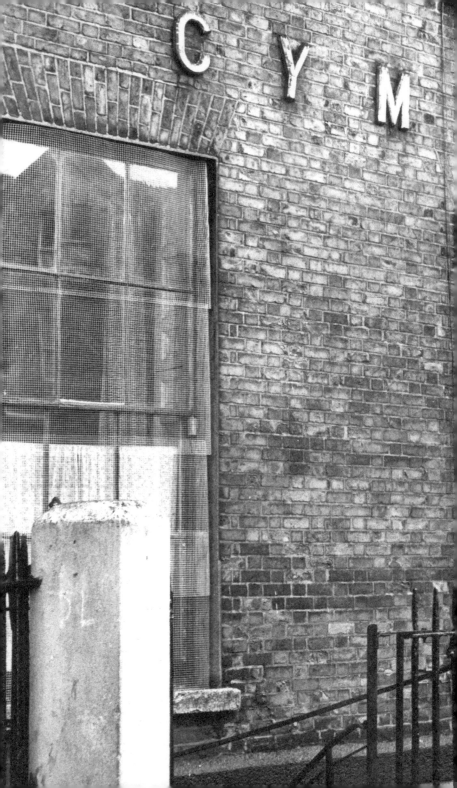

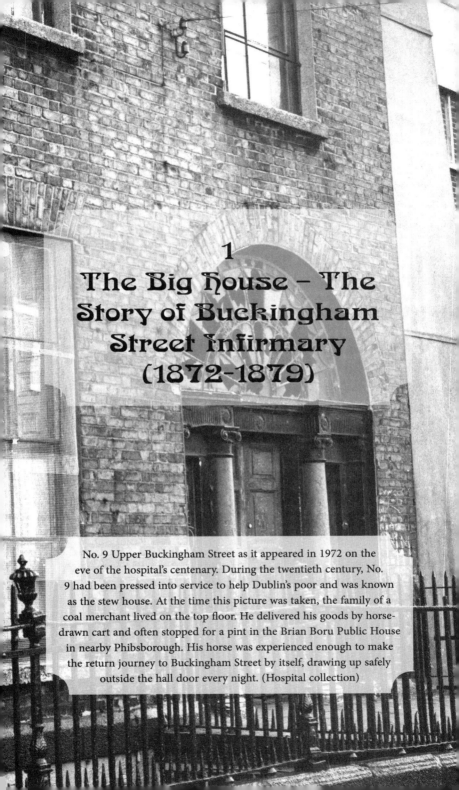

1
The Big House – The Story of Buckingham Street Infirmary (1872-1879)

No. 9 Upper Buckingham Street as it appeared in 1972 on the eve of the hospital's centenary. During the twentieth century, No. 9 had been pressed into service to help Dublin's poor and was known as the stew house. At the time this picture was taken, the family of a coal merchant lived on the top floor. He delivered his goods by horse-drawn cart and often stopped for a pint in the Brian Boru Public House in nearby Phibsborough. His horse was experienced enough to make the return journey to Buckingham Street by itself, drawing up safely outside the hall door every night. (Hospital collection)

Temple Street Hospital, now one of Ireland's best-recognised institutions, had the most humble of beginnings. It started life in a late nineteenth-century city characterised by a stark contrast between rich and poor; one in which almost half of the 250,000 inhabitants lived in cramped, single-room tenement apartments, often just streets away from their wealthy neighbours.

Disease and malnutrition were rife in the poorly-lit Georgian tenements. Rickets – a deformity of the bones – was so commonplace that it hardly attracted notice and in many cases was caused by a meagre diet, often with skimmed milk or buttermilk which was deficient in Vitamin D.[1] Many Dubliners shared single outdoor toilets which were little more than breeding grounds for flies and parasites. In the evenings they piled into crumbling rooms where typhus fever, spread by lice in their clothing, was inescapable. Outside, a charcoal-smelling fog lingered, brought on by coal fires which choked the lungs, and many babies died with no medical attention of any kind. Broken stairwells and faulty railings ensured that many more succumbed to serious injury and death.

Against this backdrop, St. Joseph's Infirmary for Children (Temple Street's forerunner) stood as a beacon of hope. Opened in November 1872, it was unlike other small, charitably run institutions because it served a specific and long-standing need – medical care for poor children in their own environment. The committee established to oversee the project met for the first time in 1871. It was led by Ellen Woodlock, a widow from Cork, and Sarah Atkinson, from Roscommon, two able women with excellent track records in charity work. Mrs Woodlock had spent some time as a novitiate with the Sisters of St Louis in France during the

1840s, but left before she completed her training.[2] Returning to Ireland, she threw herself into a number of philanthropic endeavours, including St. Joseph's Industrial Institute on Richmond Road, Fairview, which she co-founded with Sarah Atkinson in 1855.[3] The aim of the institute was to save young workhouse girls from misery and, six years later, Woodlock was the only woman to give evidence at a House of Commons select committee on poor relief in Ireland.[4]

The house they chose for their new infirmary was No. 9 Upper Buckingham Street, a large three-bay house of exceptional size. Built by Irish statesman John Beresford, it boasted massive first-floor windows and an upstairs view of the Hill of Howth.[5] Beresford's son Claudius, who lived there during the early nineteenth century, had bankrupted the family with his lavish entertainments and afterwards it passed into a succession of hands.[6]

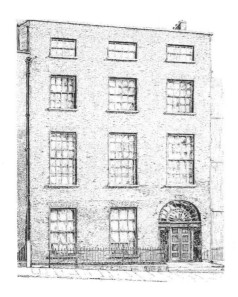

An idealised depiction of No. 9 Upper Buckingham Street from a 1972 sketch by N. Latimer. (Hospital collection)

During the summer of 1872, the painters and carpenters set to work. Beds were brought in and a wooden recess was installed at the top of the grand staircase for milk, fruit and other items. The hospital committee, which rotated on an annual basis, included two secretaries and a treasurer, the first of whom was Thomas Woodlock[7] of Uplands, Monkstown. He appealed for donations, including gifts of clothes, books and toys in order to defray the infirmary's running costs. On glancing through this list, we find pots of jam, storybooks cakes, homemade baby clothes as well as a music box from Mr Bianconi, proprietor of the famous coach company.[8]

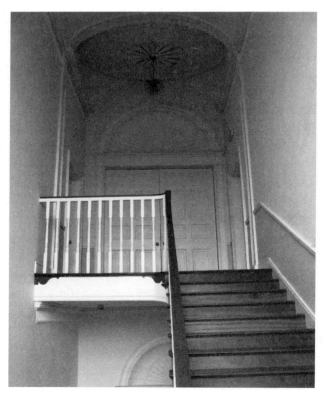

First floor landing of No. 9 Upper Buckingham Street. (Author's collection)

The Big House

By 7 November 1872, the Buckingham Street infirmary was finally ready to open its doors. The matron presided over a little coterie of nurses but in general the hospital was managed 'by women who were mothers in their own homes, and girls with the glamour of youth'.[9] They came at dinner hour to serve the food and Mrs Atkinson, spurred into charitable work by the death of her only son, aged four, also attended for several hours every day. Only patients under the age of ten were eligible for admission, however. The first was a child with spinal disease known simply to all as 'Willie'. In May 1873, the following account of his care was reported in the hospital's newly published *Tiny Bulletin*:

> He had been living in a wretched and crowded home, where five persons slept in one straw bed, and where his little brother used to kick his poor back while asleep. His first request was to be so laid in bed that he could see the beautiful statue and the flowers beside it.[10]

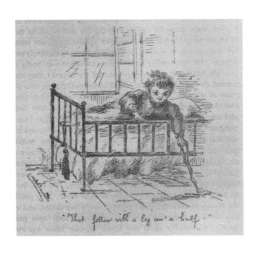

'That fellow with a leg an' a half.'

Early hospital patient from a sketch by Mary Banim. (Hospital collection)

In keeping with the Catholic ethos of the hospital (although all were accepted, regardless of denomination), a large statue of the Sacred Heart stood in the main ward and religious pictures hung on the walls. The beds had white coverlets, each trimmed with a strip of red. One of the volunteers later recalled:

> They [the patients] were often so weak that they could not stand on their feet because their parents were so poor that they could not give them food ... a poor mother might take them up on her knee and cry over them for a little while, but she had soon to put them down again and shut them up alone, and go away to her work. They were there when a friend went in, sitting on the earthen floor perhaps or among the cinders by a small spark of fire, or lying on some straw in a corner, all grimy, with their hair matted and rough, and red feverish spots burning on their wasted little cheeks. Sometimes they were coughing and crying for their mothers, sometimes quite quiet and patient, not expecting anything good to happen to them.

Apart from its inpatient work, St. Joseph's also maintained a little dispensary for outpatients. It ran every Tuesday, Thursday and Saturday for one hour in the morning but this later extended to a daily service. The entrance was in Bailey's Row, a narrow lane to the rear of the building, and applicants were asked to bring a ticket or note of recommendation from a subscriber or member of the clergy.[11] Another interesting feature of the infirmary was that it housed a lending library for the poor of the north inner city. Sometimes this was a source of comfort for mothers whose children could not be admitted on the basis of their age:

It is sad to see the poor mother turning away disappointed, with the sick child in her arms, and beautiful to observe how she will sometimes rejoice at the success of her neighbour, when her own request has been denied ... she carries away with her from the library ... a story book for the comfort of poor big Johnny at home. In this way, we can sometimes give a little out-door relief.[12]

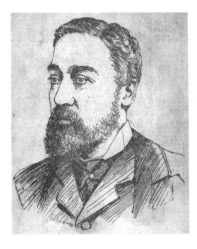

Dr Thomas More Madden as he was depicted in the *Daily Independent*, 28 October 1896.

Of the four doctors who were associated with the infirmary in its early years, the foremost was obstetrician and gynaecologist Dr Thomas More Madden. In September 1872, he had been elected as a member of the Dublin Sanitary Association, whose object was the provision of better housing conditions in the city.[13] His involvement with the infirmary served to broaden that interest and, in 1873, his children sent gifts of books, illustrated papers and toys. When fundraising concerts were held, the Madden home acted as a ticket outlet.[14]

Working alongside Madden was Dr John Francis McVeagh. The son of an excise official, McVeagh was physician to St Mary's asylum and the government female reformatory in Drumcondra. Among his achievements, he had carried out some novel experiments for the treatment of asthma and diabetes mellitus.[15]

Some of the children who attended Buckingham Street had scrofula (a kind of TB spread by unpasteurised milk), gastric disease or orthopaedic problems, but many more were simply starving. Two toddlers were so malnourished that they were 'hardly any bigger than babies', one nurse recalled. Another 'cried at the sight of food, or any vessel which might be supposed to contain it'.[16] When these children were well enough, they were dressed in donated clothes and taken to convalesce in the garden. In many cases, they were sent home in the same outfits to protect them from the cold.

The infirmary offered a brief but welcome respite from dismal tenement conditions, but in order to ensure that only the very poorest were received, ladies of the management committee took it in turns to visit the surrounding slums. There they could assess whether or not a sick child lived in comfort or poverty.

Healthy children of the middle classes were encouraged to visit the hospital on Sundays. Some were members of the 'Busy Bee Brigade', which arrived with little barrel-shaped money boxes full of pennies for the sick patients. On one occasion, they listened to a sermon given by the local priest, Father Naughton, who reminded them: 'One day poor Willie, who is lying upstairs so sick will open the door of heaven to every one of you'.[17] When a small party of children visited in 1876, their chaperone left the following pen portrait: 'The place did not look dismal at all', she wrote. 'The sun was shining in pleasantly through the chinks of cool blinds, and a number of little heads were propped up from the pillows to gaze at the visitors'. One of the guests, a girl named Sylvia, ventured over shyly to a group of patients who were playing in a corner by the window. After a few moments, they warmed to her:

One girl, taking courage, explained to the little lady that they were playing 'hospital'. They had a number of tiny wooden dolls in a box, all laid up on little heaps of rags, and tucked around, and supposed to be in bed ... Sylvia was soon busily engaged in this play, having added a pretty doll, who made so large a patient that she had to get a separate box of her own for a bed. 'Oh, but her cheeks is too rosy!' lisped a pale-faced little sprite, who was gazing rapturously at the waxen beauty. 'She isn't sick at all, but lovely and well, I'm sure'. 'That is the high fever,' explained Sylvia. 'I know when people have fever their cheeks get very red'.[18]

Fundraising was integral to Buckingham Street's success. When the infirmary first opened, it was only able to admit patients to a downstairs room. That left the entire upper part of the house vacant. Regular advertisements appeared in the *Freeman's Journal*, helped in part by the fact that the *Journal's* joint proprietor was married to Sarah Atkinson. Other appeals were printed in *The Irish Times*. They reminded readers that all of those who supported a bed or subscribed £20 or more were eligible to become a governor for life.[19] An old account book from the hospital archive chronicles donations from the 'Children of Mary' and the 'Boys' Brigade', including a number of charity sermons throughout the city.[20]

Unsurprisingly, the demands on Buckingham Street infirmary grew dramatically and during its first three and a half years up to December 1876, there were 10,000 dispensary prescriptions and over 500 admissions.[21] That put pressure on the governors, who began to run out of funds – a problem that had bedevilled some of Woodlock and Atkinson's previous endeavours. Indeed, the infirmary would certainly have had to close were it not for the fact that the two ladies had continued to maintain a strong friendship with religious orders. Mrs Woodlock had been successful in bringing the Sisters of St. Louis to County Monaghan in 1859, for instance, and when Atkinson's school for girls in Drumcondra experienced financial difficulties, she invited the Sisters of Charity to take charge.[22]

And so it was that on 2 July 1876, Buckingham Street infirmary became the nineteenth house of the Congregation of the Sisters of Charity.[23] The sisters had a long track record in healthcare, but the task they faced was not an easy one. They inherited a debt of £148 15s and one day, when a railway porter arrived with a box, the nuns had no money to pay him. On wet days, rain came through the roof and the windows were sometimes blown in. In the beginning, the sisters had to return to sleep at Vincent's Hospital on St. Stephen's Green, but after a few weeks some mattresses were brought in and they slept on those instead.[24] Shortly before Christmas 1877, they were able to attract a great deal of publicity for their new venture by encouraging the lady lieutenant to visit. She was led around the hospital by the new mother superior and took a great interest in each of the cases. Her visit, which set a long-standing annual precedent, included a gift of toys for the children.[25]

In order to get the institution on a solid footing, the sisters decided to further restrict admission to children who were suffering from acute illnesses and at the same time they substituted the name 'infirmary' for 'hospital'. On the streets outside, visitors often met children who had been treated there and Buckingham Street is remembered even today. The infirmary catered exclusively for the poor children of Dublin, but the care and attention it bestowed set a precedent for the very best in Irish paediatric hospital care. Similarly, the small sums of money donated by the Boys' Brigade and young ladies' associations, their endless hours of assistance and their enthusiasm were crucial to the hospital's success. Written 140 years ago, their letters are still imbued with real human spirit. '12 pennies for the sick children', one reads. 'Pray for mamma and for us'.

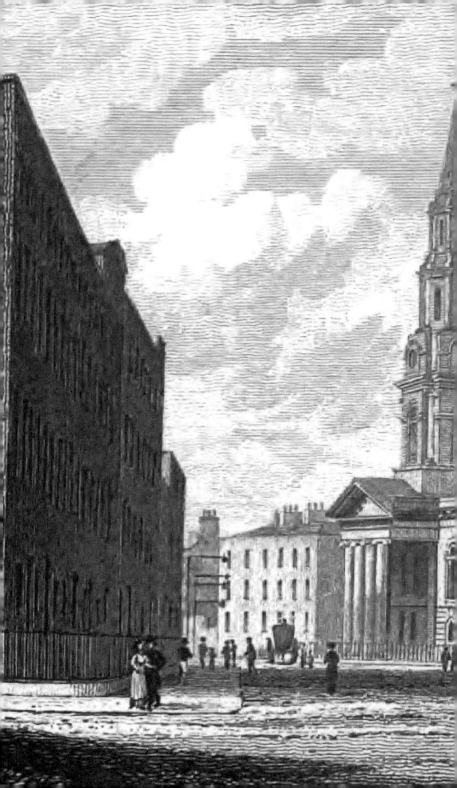

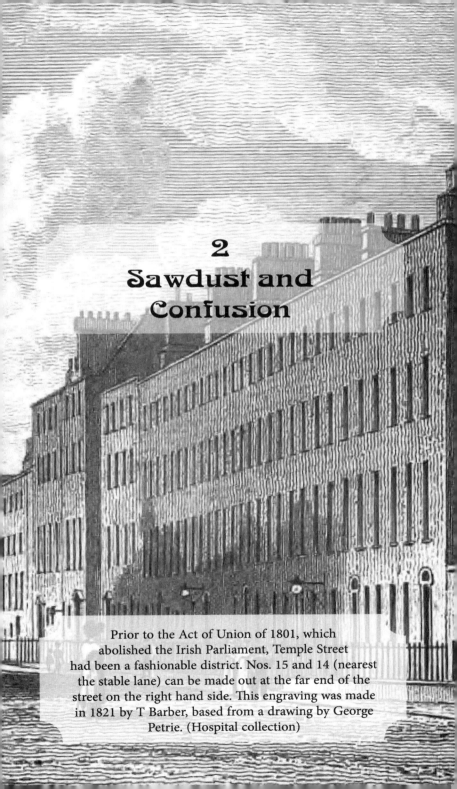

2
Sawdust and
Confusion

Prior to the Act of Union of 1801, which
abolished the Irish Parliament, Temple Street
had been a fashionable district. Nos. 15 and 14 (nearest
the stable lane) can be made out at the far end of the
street on the right hand side. This engraving was made
in 1821 by T Barber, based from a drawing by George
Petrie. (Hospital collection)

When the lease on Buckingham Street expired in 1879, a new location for the hospital had to be found. With help from a posthumous bequest from Stephen Simpson, a wealthy landowner, the sisters soon identified a suitable home for their endeavours – a handsome redbrick Georgian house at No. 15 Upper Temple Street, the former mansion of the Earl of Bellomont.[26] At that time, it was just one among many abandoned buildings in the area.

In the surrounding laneways, hundreds of tenement dwellers courted the spectres of malnutrition and sickness. In describing the scene he encountered at a house on Nerney's Court, City Analyst Charles Cameron wrote: 'no bed; sacks thrown on floor ... diet of bread and tea, no butter, bacon occasionally and cabbage Sundays'.[27] Nearby, Kelly's Row also appeared frequently in poor law reports and outbreaks of typhus and smallpox were commonplace. Likewise, in 1880, Dr John Ferguson reported to the Royal Sanitary Commission: 'I am sorry to say that in Kelly's Row, Temple-place and White's lane there are no sewers at all, and the way the surface water is carried off is down an inclined plane'.[28] The houses adjoined a dairy, a stonecutter's and even a blacksmith's, where on a weekly basis the horses from two local bakeries – Johnston Mooney & O'Brien and Kennedy's – were taken to be shod. Local author Patrick Ryan, whose childhood experience of the forge during the 1960s was probably not all that different to that of his Victorian predecessors, recalls:

As a kid going to school each morning we would stop at the forge in the lane and watch the horses being shod.

Sawdust and Confusion

It was a magical sight to see the red roaring fire, the hammer striking the red-hot shoe, the sparks flying. It was mesmerising and we were in awe until someone shouted … and the little bald blacksmith would come charging out like a mad bull out of the fires of hell! There was a mad scatter and we would be falling over each other trying to get away.[29]

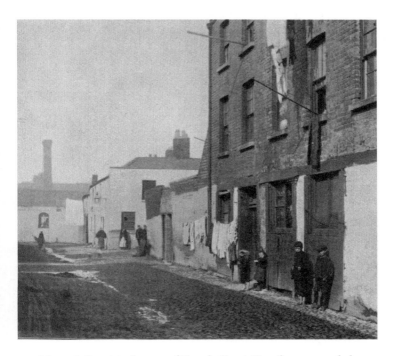

Nerney's Court to the rear of Temple Street. Heavily overcrowded, the lane was one of the poorest neighbourhoods in Dublin. Note the statue in the distance that told visitors they were in the vicinity of a hospital. (Courtesy of Dublin City Library and Archive)

Temple Street Children's Hospital

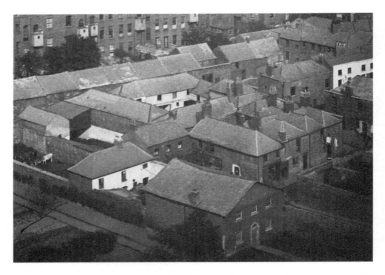

Bird's eye view of Nerney's Court taken from the clock tower of nearby St. George's Church. Note the forge on the corner which was still in operation up until the late 1950s. Some cattle can be seen in a yard outside the hospital garden. Mountjoy Square stands in the distance. (Courtesy of Royal Society of Antiquaries)

Shortly after taking over the running of Temple Street Hospital, the Sisters of Charity began to make forays into the surrounding area – an effort that exposed them to the very illnesses they were trying to treat.[30] Along Nerney's Court and Kelly's Row, their habits could be heard rattling until they reached a particular darkened stairwell or basement. More often than not, the scene was heart-rending – the waxen face of a deceased parent surrounded by candles or a malnourished child lying on dirty straw. In December 1896, the Jesuit *Irish Monthly* – always a strong supporter of the hospital – printed a short drama written by Rosa Mulholland (Lady Gilbert) which described 'two angels' visiting a poor home near Temple Street with 'no bread upon the shelf'. As late as June 1923, one student nurse who had been educated in Edinburgh was surprised to see the 'dirty condition of children on admission' and between times, many families continued to depend on the hospital's 'silent service' for support. The hospital's Annual Report for 1933 put it thus:

> Only he who observes those groups assembling at the Out-Patients' Department each evening to receive bread, tea and sugar, meat, clothing, and those little tickets which mean the open sesame to milk and coal can realise that the dispensary is not finished when the doctors leave ... then there is the whispered plea to the Sister in the ward of the black-shawled mother who is taking her cured child back to the same squalid surroundings and unthinkable hardship which but a few weeks ago had sent it in an ambulance to the hospital door.[31]

Some of the poorest children were taken to Temple Street simply for nourishment. 'Each little child before going home gets a hot lunch of ... bread and soup, Irish stew or rice', one nun wrote. 'The little ones who attend our dispensary are wretchedly poor. It is hopeless to try and cure them without feeding them ... one of our greatest difficulties was providing spoons which rapidly disappeared until we arranged that each child should bring her own.'[32]

Although the house to which these children were admitted has now changed beyond recognition, traces of it still remain. Today's replica stucco ceiling at the entrance to No. 15 masks the location of an old winding staircase whose banister swept up over the hallway fireplace onto the first floor or *piano nobile,* where in times past the master of the house entertained his visitors. There, the main reception rooms were decorated in a neo-classical style and were accessible through doors arranged in a row or *enfilade.*

The first floor also had an impressive dividing screen, comprising scagliola-coated columns and pilasters decorated with Corinthian capitals.[33] On the ground floor, there was no dividing corridor between the 'front' and 'back' parlours. Instead, the two rooms formed one large compartment, probably divided by a wooden partition.[34] Throughout the house, the floorboards were made of pitch pine – a North American import much favoured for its rot-resistance.

In order to prepare these rooms for the arrival of their little guests, the sisters turned them over to an army of workmen. One lady lent some curtains from her drawing room and others sent candlesticks and vases. A Protestant gentleman even robbed his greenhouse of its nicest flowers for the altar. As the builders downed tools each evening, the sisters made a home for themselves in the old tack and harness room of the stables amid 'sawdust and confusion' and 'having barred the doors and windows with any furniture or planks about the place, went to bed'.[35]

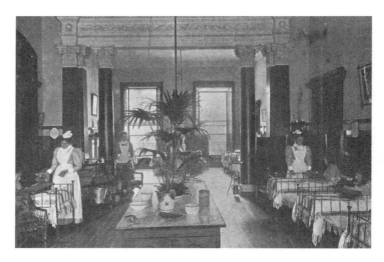

St. Agnes' Ward, c.1890. (Hospital collection)

By day, the stables looked out onto a large and overgrown garden – once part of the Barley Fields where the 1798 insurgents convened. The sisters introduced chickens so that they could have fresh eggs and they planted vegetables and made a play area for convalescent children. Inside, the kitchen, with its space for a larder, stores servants' rooms and patient wardrobes, sprang to life once again and coal was delivered into the great bunkers under the street just as it had during the days of the Earl of Bellomont.

By 17 June 1879, the hospital was ready to open its doors to the public. It boasted twenty-one beds and was staffed by the same doctors who had attended Buckingham Street. Many continued to hold posts at other hospitals, but they were unable to claim a professional salary for their work. As a result, nearby North Frederick Street, with its string of private practices, became the 'Harley Street' of Dublin.

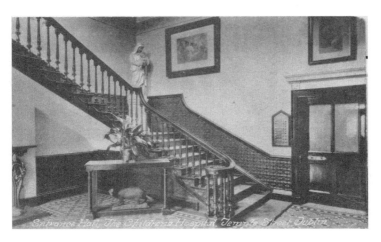

Entrance hall at Temple Street, c.1900. Note the tessellated tile pattern, some of which is still in evidence today. The staircase has long since been removed. (Hospital collection)

While the sisters busied themselves with making the old mansion a hospital, a private householder continued to live next door in a slightly smaller Georgian redbrick – once home to Charles Stewart Parnell and his family.[36] In 1881, he decided to relinquish the property in favour of 'a good Farm of Pasture Land, near a railway station, within thirty or forty miles of Dublin'.[37] The sisters recognised their chance to enlarge the hospital and they seized it with both hands.[38] On Sunday, 3 February 1884, some friends of Temple Street convened in its empty drawing room with the purpose of establishing a hospital 'Extension Fund'. The *Irish Monthly* remarked that 'the new house is a fine one, with large rooms easily convertible into delightful wards for small patients in cribs; but at present its only furniture consists of an old sofa and some feathers!'[39]

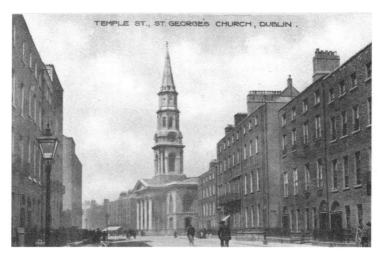

TEMPLE ST., ST. GEORGE'S CHURCH, DUBLIN.

Postcard of Temple Street Hospital in 1931. Note the original red-brick facade and balcony. In 1940, a new plaster render was put in place.
(Hospital collection)

When work got underway the following year, it was of sufficient importance to merit a mention in London's *Building News and Engineering Journal*, the editors commenting that the new addition was to include a convalescent ward and parlour on the ground floor, a general ward with a bathroom on the first floor and two wards on the second level.[40] An entrance was broken through on every floor in order to join the houses into one and, understandably, the outlay was significant. Fortunately, the sisters were thrifty enough to let out the old coach house and stables at the rear of No. 14. Later, they noted in the annals that 'the incoming rent almost suffices to pay all the ground rent of the entire hospital'.[41] Temple Street was now ready to begin its life-saving work in earnest.

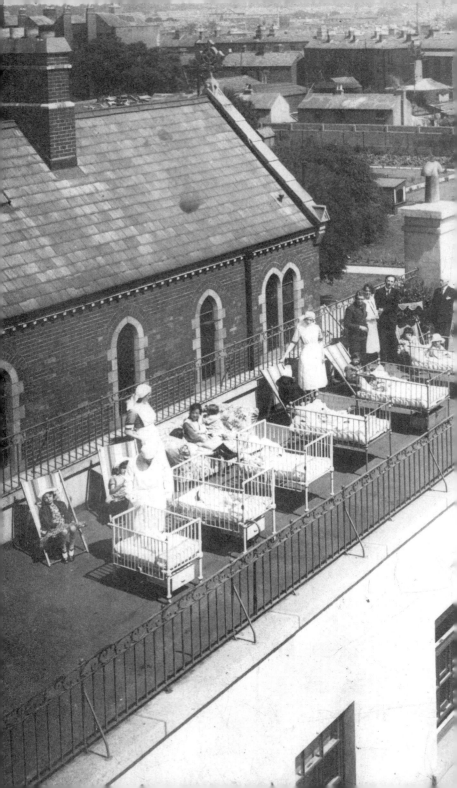

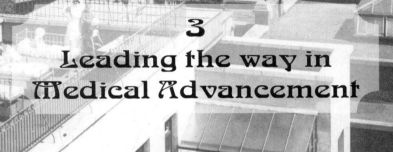

3
Leading the way in
Medical Advancement

A group of children from St. Patrick's Ward benefit
from sunshine or 'heliotherapy', c.1932. The cots had
green, adjustable shades. (Hospital collection)

Temple Street Children's Hospital

During Temple Street's early years, only patients between the ages of two and ten were eligible for admission. On arrival, they were issued with a new set of clothes and, regardless of sex, their hair was cropped short to limit the spread of lice. Unlike today, the wards in which they slept were more like large nurseries and many remained for a month or more – far longer than would be considered usual today. Recalling one memorable visit in 1892, Mary Banim, the daughter of a novelist, wrote that the children were kept 'in rows of snug cribs ranged around the walls, a number of little girls are keeping holiday, some in bed, some up and dressed … there was a real nun … holding a small baby on the prancing rocking-horse, laughing the while as if her own turn were coming next'.[42]

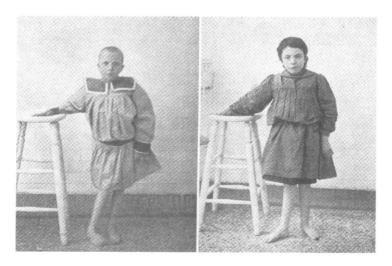

Rickets was a particularly prevalent problem during the early years of the twentieth century. These two children were patients in 1911. The boy on the left would appear to have had his head shaved – perhaps as a treatment for lice. (Hospital collection)

Leading the way in Medical Advancement

Banim delighted in speaking to the patients, one particular favourite being a shy five-year-old named Lily, whom she described as 'an old sufferer'. In order to treat her spinal deformity, Lily was obliged to lie, strapped day and night, in bed with heavy weights attached to her legs. An adjacent sliding table was covered with 'whole families of dolls and their peculiar belongings and a box full of scraps of coloured stuffs, out of which "the dolls' dressmaker" selects the materials for costumes'. In another corner, a nun cared for a three-year-old child 'whose death from bronchitis was expected all through the night, but who the Sister says they now trust will pull through'.

The sixty children were usually put to sleep at six o'clock each evening, but some, by virtue of their adult responsibilities, could hardly be described as such. 'Miss Kate' (aged ten) was obliged to support her mother and three younger sisters after her father's death. Another girl named Mary (aged twelve) explained that she received her injuries while preparing supper for her father who was out at work. 'My legs and hips were nearly scalded off', she explained, 'and sure, wasn't it well I'd just laid the child down out of my arms!'

At the time of Banim's visit, there were also several Irish-speaking patients at the hospital. One boy, whose father had been drowned in a storm the previous winter, had been taken there from his Aran island home by his grandmother. She came to Dublin 'dressed in her island costume of red petticoat, dark gown, white or plaid shawl', Banim wrote, 'and on her feet "pampoaties" [*sic*] or cow-hide sandals'. Afterwards, she wrote to the nuns, eliciting a promise that if her grandson could not be cured, he would return to 'sleep in the old church-yard where the sea rolls up almost to the very graves'.

Every day, healthy children were encouraged to visit but only parents were allowed to call on Sundays. One particular bed was paid for solely through donations from the pupils of nearby Loreto Convent, North Great George's Street. Other children were encouraged to donate their pennies or toys. Girls were particularly sought after for their sewing skills and, on request, the superioress was prepared to post clothing patterns to them.

By 1884, the number of children attending the dispensary at Temple Street had doubled and in the same year, some 650 children attended with scrofula alone. In 1882, German bacteriologist Robert Koch discovered that TB was an infectious disease, but it took some time for this to become widely accepted and it was not acknowledged as a significant factor in the city's high death rate until 1900.

Many of the doctors who practised at Temple Street had learned their trade during an era in which 'Heroic Medicine' predominated. It included practices such as intestinal purging (with calomel), bloodletting (venesection), vomiting (tartar emetic), profuse sweating (diaphoretics) and blistering. Although such methods had begun to fall out of favour by the 1880s, a number of them continued to prevail. Until the early 1900s, for instance, the hospital continued to buy large quantities of leeches for blood-letting.[43] Another generally held theory was that infection was transported by a noxious gas or miasma and, depending on the wind, the hospital windows often had to be closed due to the smell from the adjacent piggery. The standard practice at Temple Street was to soak bedclothes and doors with chloride of lime and Condy's fluid as it was believed that fires burning in the wards would draw up the 'miasma' through the chimney. 'A very small child was in a comfortable chair by a blazing fire', *Irish Times* correspondent Lucy Leonard wrote in December 1893, 'but had a cough and was so sleepy and cross that she would not even look at us'.[44]

Sepsis was the 'pestilence that walketh in darkness' in the dingy, overcrowded wards of large hospitals. Four illnesses flared up with such frequency that they came to be known collectively as 'hospital disease' – erysipelas, septicaemia, pyaemia and acute gangrene. As a result, very little abdominal surgery was performed and there was no understanding about how viruses were transmitted. The rate of congenital deformities of the nervous system was higher in Dublin than elsewhere in the country, with 380 cases of hydrocephalus (water on the brain) seen at Temple Street in 1884 alone. Most of these cases were managed palliatively since the techniques necessary to drain and re-circulate cerebral spinal fluid had not yet been devised. On 20 August 1887, the *British Medical Journal* summarised the findings of a paper given by Dr More Madden in which he attributed the root cause of the 'increasing prevalence of cerebral disease' (including meningitis, cephalitis, headaches, sleeplessness and neuroses of all kinds) to 'the daily increasing educational pressure now brought to bear on children from a very early age'. In this, he was supported by Dr Charles Cameron, who added that children of the poorer classes were unable to apply themselves at school due to malnutrition.[45]

But despite these difficulties, the removal of children from the wards of general adult hospitals was regarded as a positive step. Disregarding infectious patients (who were cared for at the Cork Street Fever Hospital), it is a remarkable fact that in a city where one-third of the total deaths were attributable to children under five, the mortality rate at Temple Street prior to 1900 remained under four percent.

Anatomical knowledge had reached quite an advanced stage when the hospital first opened its doors. It was of some assistance in trauma cases, many of which resulted from defective tenement railings or stairwells, but there were no X-rays and everything depended on touch and observation. Until the new operating theatre was opened by the lord lieutenant in 1904, it was standard practice for surgeons to operate on the ward, daylight permitting, with help from a trainee house surgeon who earned his living from an 'assistant's fee'.[46] Nevertheless, relatively few cases could be performed with any degree of safety and appendicitis, which affected as many as one in ten of the population, was almost always left to take its own course in the hope that an abscess, amenable to drainage, might develop.

By the 1880s, it was no longer acceptable to operate on conscious, albeit mechanically restrained children. They harboured 'an expectation of something worse than what is actually felt, and generally a deficiency of resolution, that renders it impossible for them to be sufficiently quiet'.[47] Anaesthesia was the solution, but until the introduction of endotracheal intubation the airway could not be maintained with safety and as a result most surgical procedures lasted no longer than twenty minutes. Intra-operatively, many surgeons were obliged to improvise by making their own surgical instruments and even provide their own rubber gloves. Mr John Shanley, one of Temple Street's earliest paediatric surgeons (1895–1975), recalled that:

> Not only were there no antibiotics or blood transfusions, but parenteral fluids [saline with glucose, electrolytes, etc] were usually given subcutaneously or intraperitoneally, both of which must have been very painful to the patient; the anaesthesia of that time would now be considered quite primitive; usually it was the 'rag and bottle' method.[48]

Post-operatively, patients were treated with a regimen of beef tea and aromatic sulphuric acid for shock – a mixture of ginger, oil of cinnamon and alcohol. Ice packs were commonly applied. Grains of opium were administered to alleviate pain or, in the case of babies, judicious spoonfuls of laudanum – a brandy-based tincture.[49] While there was perhaps less concern that children might become narcotised, doctors in paediatric practice were nevertheless alive to the dangers of administering a harmful dose.

Although other techniques such as clinical thermometry, chemical tests and auscultation were still quite new, as early as 1877 H. MacNaughton in his *Clinical Teaching in Hospitals* recommended that students attending the sick should carry a stethoscope, clinical thermometer, pocket measure, scissors, forceps, probe, small scalpel, lancet, silk and silver wire and litmus paper as well as a pocket urinary test apparatus. Another part of every doctor's kit was the methylated spirit lamp which, unlike paraffin, did not give off an unpleasant odour and helped to disinfect spoons, needles and other items.

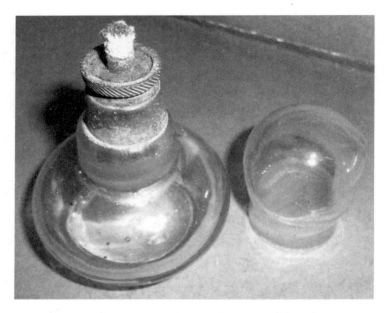

This spirit lamp burner was used at Temple Street and dates from 1890–1910. Fuelled by methylated spirits, such lamps were used to sterilise medicine spoons, measures and needles. (Author's collection)

In its favour, Temple Street Hospital was well equipped with medical staff. By comparison, the County and City of Cork Hospital for Women and Children had just one consultant surgeon and five medical officers, despite its comparable number of inpatients. The complement at Temple Street included physicians as well as dental, resident and assistant surgeons and children were soon being referred from all over the country due to its favourable patient-doctor ratio. In part, this was assured by the large influx of students from the city's medical schools, of which there were three – the Royal College of Surgeons, Trinity College and the Catholic University School in Cecilia Street. The Children's Hospital maintained an especially close relationship with the latter, with Dr More Madden sitting on the governing board of Cecilia Street after it was brought under the supervision of the Education Endowment Commission in 1891.

Although hospital positions went unpaid, it was often considered essential to obtain a post in one, particularly if one's career and reputation was to be established. Nevertheless, a doctor still could not qualify on the basis of his paediatric experience alone; he needed to spend a period of time in a general adult hospital.[50] Between times, he had to supplement his income through private practice. Those junior doctors who wished to secure training posts usually had to visit each of these clinics in turn in the hope of securing an interview. Esther Bridgeman (ninety-two), whose son was treated for asthma by Dr Kidney during the 1950s, recalls:

> I used to have to pay a guinea each time I visited him in Merrion Square which was £1.1. The treatment then was that I was given this thing with a rubber piece on the bottom; the same as you would see on a bike. I used to have to open it up, put the medication in and squeeze it until it went into his throat. 'The one thing I want you to do, never once mention A.S.T.H.M.A.' Dr Kidney said. 'The less they know about it the better.' You see, he thought the child was likely to act up once you put a name on the condition.[51]

From 1886, students were obliged to pass examinations in midwifery and surgery as well as medicine, and towards the end of the century the period of time they spent as undergraduates increased. In the morning they attended Temple Street's outpatient

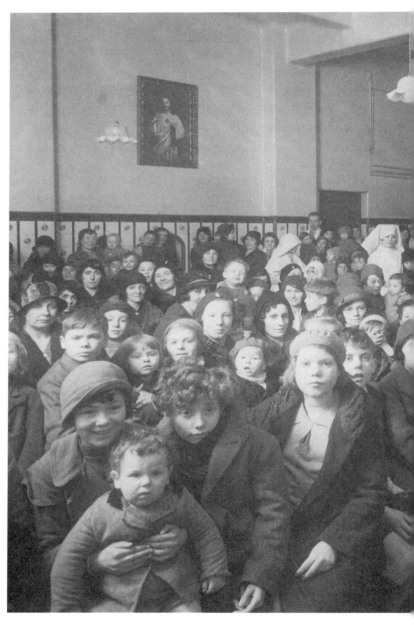

Outpatient department at Temple Street, 1930. This building has be[

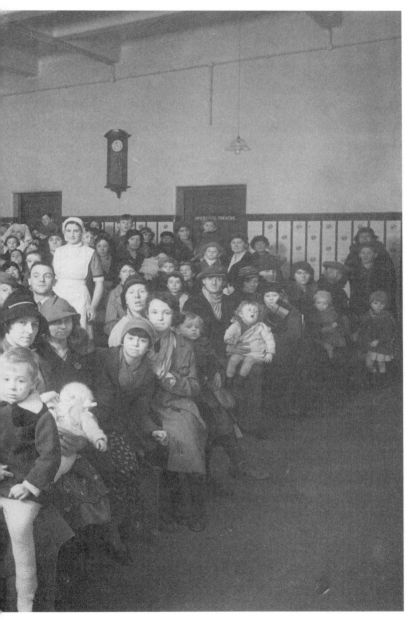

)us use since it was first opened a century ago. (Hospital collection)

department where, until a new referrals system came into effect as a result of the Health Act of 1953, it was common to see a hundred or so patients at a single session. 'Youthful license and ... ungentlemanly frivolity' was to be avoided and since there were no sub-specialities, students helped the consultant to treat everything from broken bones to sore throats – occasionally running the gauntlet of an escaped pig in the waiting room or taking a child to the adjacent blacksmith to have a piece of metal removed from a finger or limb.[52] The afternoon left them free to attend lectures and dissections.

The absence of paediatrics as a topic on the medical examination meant that only a small number of students accompanied the hospital consultants on their rounds. This came as a source of regret to Dr John McVeagh, who in November 1889 stressed to them 'the importance of devoting a part of their time to the study of the peculiarities of disease as observed in children'. A half century later, students still had to provide all of their own instruments as well as their white coats. Despite the establishment of the *British Journal of Disease of Children* in 1904 and the inauguration of the Irish Paediatric Association, there were still only a handful of paediatricians in the British Isles.

Medical care, however, continued to progress. By the middle of the twentieth century, serious cases of rickets were thankfully becoming rare and malnutrition was not seen as often in paediatric practice. Nevertheless, there was still unacceptable poverty in the heart of Dublin. Babies continued to arrive at the hospital carrying their own weight in clothing in order to stave off the cold. In 1949, one child was even admitted with thirteen layers on his chest, including a piece of carpet.[53] Dr Livinia Meenan, who came to Temple Street as a house physician for six months in 1952, recalls:

> There was deprivation in those post-war years but I never saw anything like the poverty in the inner city. There were high levels of infectious diseases – in particular measles and meningitis and many accident cases. I recall children coming in who had tried to ride on the backs of carts. They described it as 'scuttin'. You would be told, 'Ah he fell and I gave him a dose of castor oil. Sure, the poor child.'

When taking a medical history, a child's mother would often give the father's occupation as 'casual'. Many mothers came to A&E simply because their infants wouldn't sleep and they wanted somebody to talk to. Dr Meenan's abiding memory of that time is of being constantly on her feet: 'I remember early one summer morning when the sun had just come up. I saw no point in going back to bed so I went to Mass instead. The nuns all filed silently into the chapel wearing their long cloaks – it was almost a medieval sight.'[54]

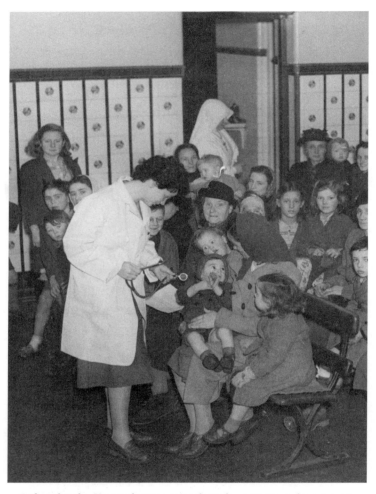

Left and right: Young doctors at work in the outpatient department,
c.1940. They had to provide their own white coats and stethoscopes.
(Hospital collection).

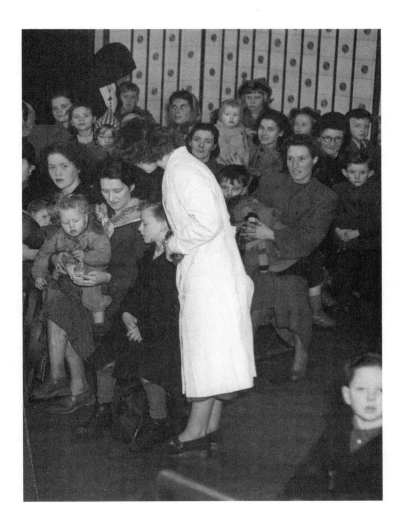

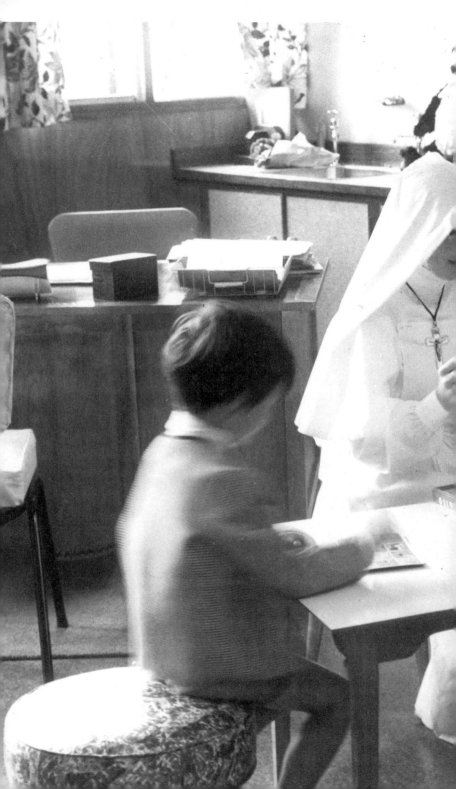

4

The Convent Community

A nun at play with hospital patients, c.1960.
(Hospital collection)

R eligious vocation went hand in hand with hospital life at Temple Street. The young nuns, whose convent was on the top floor, worked on a daily basis to fulfil the Sisters of Charity motto, *Caritas Christi Urgent Nos* (The love of Christ moves us forward).[55] Every ward was under their care and they helped to train the nurses as well as assist in surgical cases.[56] Oftentimes the cry of a child in the ward below at night would cause one of them to appear, lantern in hand, to lend a soothing touch or a kindly voice. The affection in which they held their young charges is evident from their letters and papers.

Nevertheless, the hospital could not operate on sentiment alone. Discipline was the order of the day and the arrival of visitors was usually heralded via a gong that hung at the bottom of the main staircase. Each nun had her own signal. The domestic orderly might strike once for the mother superior and twice for the sister ministress – a sound that could be heard right through the house. On one memorable occasion, retired staff member Michael Fielding recalls that a new porter in training got the code mixed up and instead of banging out four gongs and then five, just kept going:

> As the gongs went on and on, the nurses on the wards started to ring the switchboard *en-masse* because they thought it meant a fire alarm. At the same time, three or four black-habited nuns ran out of the chapel and down the stairs. Pat was still banging away by the time I reached him. 'Stop!' I shouted. 'What's going on?' 'You said gong 45 times', he answered, 'and that's what I'm doing.'[57]

The Convent Community

The sister ministress had her office in the front hall and was responsible for the welfare of her community. The mother superior, whose room was directly opposite, handled the daily running of the hospital. At intervals, they adjourned to one of the two community rooms where they mingled with other sisters trained in healthcare. There was a second community room on the lower level for those nuns who worked in the laundry and kitchen. Such work could sometimes take its toll, however, and in October 1924, the annals record that Sister M. Giles Mooney had to be changed to house works owing to a 'sharp attack of asthma'.[58]

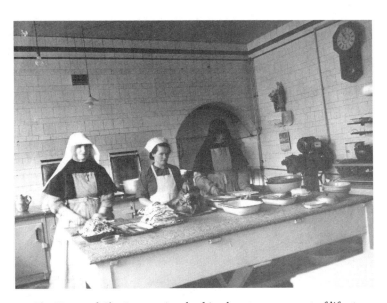

The Sisters of Charity were involved in almost every aspect of life at Temple Street. Here, two nuns help a member of the household staff to prepare lunch. Note the meat ready to be carved. In later years, this kitchen was placed under the supervision of Sr. Gilbert. (Hospital collection)

Although Temple Street Hospital was non-sectarian, it continued to maintain a Catholic ethos. The little patients were woken once a week to receive communion and the hospital echoed to the tinkle of the chaplain's bell. The hospital annals also record occasional death-bed conversions to Catholicism. 'Sometimes too', the sisters noted, 'the children (who if Catholics are instructed and prepared for the Sacraments) on their return to their homes become unconscious apostles, reminding father and mother of long-forgotten truths and long neglected practices'.[59]

In the early years, the sisters used the front and back parlour as a chapel but when the hospital was expanded in 1883, the new hall cut nine feet off their sanctuary, making it too small to be of any use. Having agreed that it was 'not conducive to a spirit of prayer', they decided to build a new chapel on the site of the billiard room to the rear of No. 14.[60] The annals record that:

> Funds not being sufficient, the Rectress, Sr M. Barnabas Delaney, hesitated to commence the building, but agreed with the community to begin a novena to St John the Evangelist, asking him, if it was the Will of God that the chapel should be built, to send a sum of £500 immediately, and they would take it as a sign that it was his Will and would dedicate the chapel to St Joseph and St John. At the end of the novena Mother Rectress went to tell Reverend Mother that she thought it much better not to go in for the building, as means were not forthcoming. However, before she had spoken on the subject … she said to Mother Rectress, 'Do you know, the Cardinal has just sent me £500 for you?' It

was a comforting and direct answer to prayer, but as the old saying goes, 'Much would have more'. When the community heard of it they only regretted that they had not asked for £2000 instead of £500.[61]

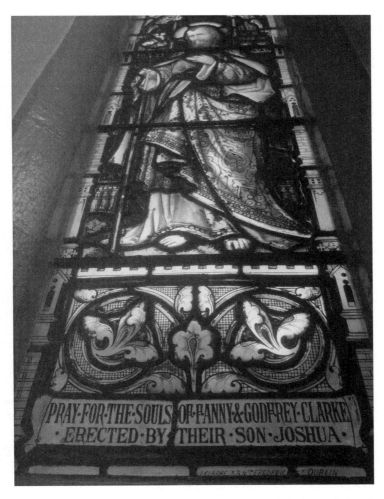

This stained glass window was erected in the sacristy of the hospital chapel to the memory of Fanny and Godfrey Clarke by their son Joshua, father of the famous Harry Clarke. (Author's collection)

Once the chapel had been consecrated, the sisters attended Mass there every morning, dressed in their long choir cloaks. Mary Threadgold (Sr Thomas Aquinas), who started at the hospital as a young postulant in 1957, recalls:

> At that time, the chapel had stalls along the walls and benches down the middle. We used to attend Mass every morning at 7am. The Jesuits from Belvedere College were our chaplains and student nurses would join us for Mass sometimes. In the 1970s, we had Vespers at 5.30pm. A couple of the household or domestic staff as they were called then would join us on Sunday evenings, having rehearsed beforehand with Sr Francis Regis, our organist.[62]

Later, offices replaced vespers and religious observance was expected of other staff too – particularly the nurses. During the angelus, work on the wards was temporarily halted.

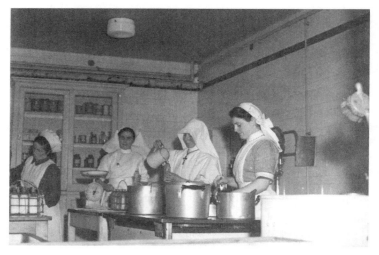

Preparing bottles in the milk kitchen, c.1930. (Hospital collection)

The Convent Community

In 1895, a devotion of St. Anthony's Bread was established at Temple Street through the efforts of a nun from the Sisters of Mercy and, two years later, the Association of St Anthony of Padua started a fund to help local children and their families. It drew much of its income from donations, but by far the most important source of funding came from *St. Anthony's Annals* – a popular hospital-produced magazine which had a monthly circulation of 11,000 by the late 1890s. The annals helped to bring the sisters' good work to an international audience and copies were sent as far afield as America, India, Africa and Australia.[63] Bert Cobbe (seventy-seven), who worked for the Antonian Press during the 1950s, recalls:

> Billy was the main man in there – he kind of ran the whole place. We used to do rosary beads, prayer books and calendars. The books had silver on the front. I used to be sent off on a bike to deliver to the Catholic shop on Cathedral Street and Adam and Eve's Church on Merchant's Quay. Sure the load of books used to be higher than the basket on the bike.[64]

The religious mission undertaken by the Sisters of Charity also extended to the surrounding community. In July 1964, the hospital almoner, Sr Francis Regis, wrote to Archbishop John Charles McQuaid to ask him whether they might extend their annual retreat day for poor mothers to the fathers on the basis that 'their example in their homes leaves much to be desired'.[65] Sr Francis Ignatius Fahy recalls:

> For some hours on a Sunday, it was possible for us to visit homes within walking distance of the hospital. We

might follow up on a particular patient or offer support and encouragement to other people who lived alone or who had become isolated for one reason or other. From time to time, outings or parties were organised. Over the years, two of these occasions became annual events. We held a Christmas party for the mothers as well as a retreat day which was usually held on a Sunday in late summer. It proved to be so popular that it was decided to extend it to the fathers. A lot of planning went into it and the regular home visiting provided an opportunity to encourage people to attend. At first, they came from the immediate neighbourhood but this changed as new estates opened up in places like Finglas and Coolock.

For the retreat days, the outpatients department was transformed into a chapel and an altar was brought into the main hall which was decorated for the occasion with flowers and plants. The adjoining rooms were also pressed into service as a sacristy and confessional. For the mothers who attended the Christmas party or retreat Sunday, the opportunity to have their meals served to them and to sit down and eat them undisturbed was a rare treat and one that they looked forward to during the course of the year. The food was beautifully prepared and served from the hospital kitchen. Porters, nurses and secretarial staff assisted and all was done with a spirit of generosity and enthusiasm that added much to the enjoyment of and popularity of those days. [66]

Although the religious community at Temple Street was quite young and vibrant in its early years, it was clear that the sisters also needed help. Around 1900, the mother general (the head of the order) consented to their request to start a day school in doll and dressing-making.[67] Afterwards, in 1904, they established a school of domestic economy and a teacher or instructress, certified by the Department of Agricultural and Technical Instruction, was appointed.[68] A letter dated 14 April 1915 shows that the sisters had employed a teacher to begin lessons in cookery and 'housewifery'. Many of the girls were quite poor, but with the advantage of training they were able to take up employment elsewhere. Bridget Dempsey from County Westmeath remembered:

> When my sister was very ill one time, my father, who was a small farmer, had to go at two o'clock in the morning with her on the motor bicycle. She had appendicitis and he used to come up after that to visit her. My father knew all the nuns and the head matron. The recession was on that time and you couldn't get a job. When I was only about sixteen, he talked to them about starting me in the hospital. 'The girls are all young', he used to say, 'and when they grow up they'll put them in for nursing'. I was put on the baby ward in St. Patrick's and they had me doing the hall door as well. Sometimes I used to help in outpatients and I was down in St. Bridget's where the tonsil cases were. There was a gong in the hall and you used to have to ring that if there was a visitor coming in ... you had to do the wards, down on your hands – polishing and dusting and then we went to Mass. [69]

That same year, the nuns started a night school at Temple Street for boys between fourteen and eighteen years of age. A male teacher taught them reading, writing and arithmetic and many of the pupils were brought through to confirmation. 'A few of them had never made their first confession,' one of the sisters recalled. 'It was wonderful to see how anxious they were to secure the sacraments.'[70]

During the 1920s, the sisters were able to expand this community-based work through the help of St. Anthony's Baby Club, whose previous premises were on Granby Lane.[71] Many of the young mothers from the surrounding tenements lacked essential skills in childcare or home management and the club, which took up residence in the hospital outpatient department around 1926, aimed to fill that gap. Chaired by a voluntary lady president with medical input from Dr John Shanley, it invited ladies to attend with their babies on weekday evenings. There they received lessons in cookery and needlework and were given clothes and basic supplies such as cod-liver oil and Virol (a malt extract). Every week, the 'little mothers' paid money towards a coal club as well as a Christmas fund. Between times, Mrs Sheridan, from her home cottage adjacent to the A&E department, gave them milk powder through a hatch in one of her downstairs windows. One local recalls:

> I remember we had to walk through that lane to collect the infant aid milk with the cardboard inserts in the top of the bottles. There was one particular goat that seemed to take a dislike to my grandmother because he used to put his head down and run at her. Thankfully she was light on her feet at the time … me gran that is; not the goat.[72]

With such support, the sisters were able to continue their vital life-saving work, symbolised by the statue of Our Lady on St.

Anthony's Lane. Every evening, Mrs Sheridan used to walk out with a long taper, her young grandson William in tow, and light the lamp. During foggy nights, it shone out as a beacon of hope – a sign that help was near at hand.

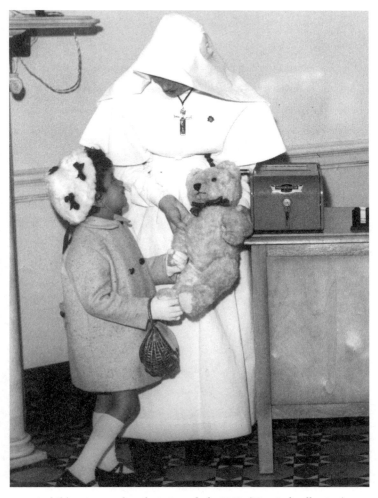

A child arrives at the admissions desk, 1960. (Hospital collection)

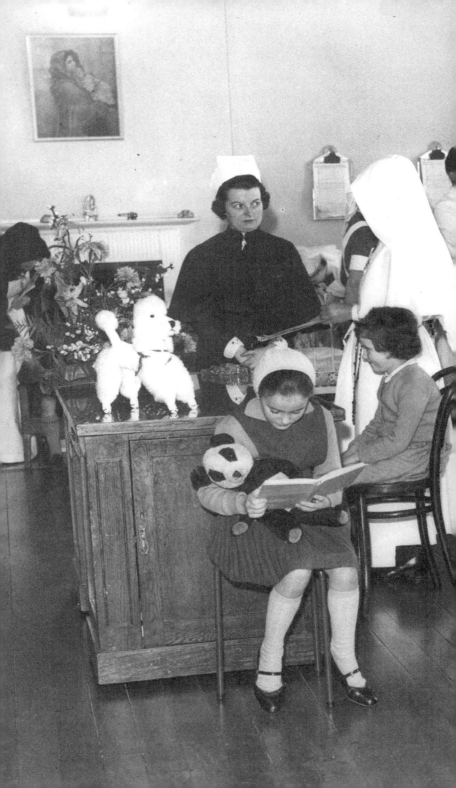

5
Field of Honey –
Fundraising at Temple
Street

Photograph of a busy ward at Temple Street, c.1960,
taken as part of a fundraising drive for the hospital. All
of the toys seen here were donated. (Hospital collection)

Fundraising was an ever-present issue for the Children's Hospital in its early days. Apart from a modest Dublin Corporation grant, there was little or no state help and since most of those who attended Temple Street were poor, inpatient fees provided a limited stream of revenue (such monies meeting just three percent of the running costs). The Association of Charities, based in Molesworth Street, ran a cooperative scheme that encouraged benevolent organisations to work together. These included the 'Police-Aided Children's Clothing Society', 'Church of Ireland Clergy Widows and Orphan's Society' and 'Sisters of Charity School' in Gardiner Street, which gave breakfast to the area's poor children every morning. Directories and newspapers were another important outlet for Temple Street Hospital because it could advertise for donations in them. In addition, *The Irish Times* and its 'League of Kindness' paid for a cot, as did the nearby Loreto convent. Nevertheless, despite such efforts, the hospital could not have existed in its early years without the support of such Irish notaries as Charles Bianconi, the famous stagecoach maker, and author and playwright Oscar Wilde.

It soon became apparent that despite their help, a more formal fundraising arrangement was needed. In response, the Moy Mell Children's Guild was inaugurated in 1896. It took its name from a Gaelic name for heaven, meaning 'Field of Honey' – a place where everyone grows young and never ages. In launching the guild, its first president, Countess Cadogan, made the following impassioned plea:

In the Children's Hospital there are a large number of poor little patients, who are sick and suffering, and I want you to help them. It is always very sad to see a little child suffer pain and sickness, even when a loving mother, a kind nurse and a skilful doctor are doing everything possible to lessen the suffering. But it is far, far sadder to know, that there are many children ill and helpless, some of whom have careless or even cruel parents, and others, too, whose mothers, with all their affection, are too poor to provide their little ones with the relief and comfort they want so badly.[73]

The response was enthusiastic and soon collection boxes began to appear in homes and businesses all over Ireland. The rules of admission stated that each little guild member had to pay a yearly entrance fee of six pence. Boys and girls were encouraged to donate toys and money or make garments for their unfortunate bed-bound peers. Girls gave two items of clothing and boys sent two toys or a money order in December. Children under seven could also take part by collecting pennies for the children's guild cot.

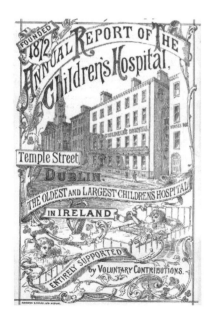

As this lavishly-illustrated annual report from 1898 clearly demonstrates, Temple Street depended on donations for its existence. (Hospital collection)

Every year, Dubliners eagerly awaited the arrival of a fundraising bazaar that was held in the grounds of the Rotunda Hospital. The gardens were lit with electric lighting, flags and bunting and people thronged to the various tents, marquees and merry-go-rounds. Against a background of brass band music, they took a turn at the swing boats and shooting galleries or had their fortune read by a clairvoyant. One novel feature during the 1890s was the cinematograph – an early precursor of the film reel. In 1893, the fête even featured a performance by the Grand Continental Circus. When some of the artistes realised that the sickest of the children could not attend, they visited the wards in person.

In an effort to bring the work of the hospital to an international audience, the sisters wrote to Maria Christina, Queen Regent of Spain, in 1897 to ask her whether she would allow her son to become a patron of the Moy Mell guild. Alphonso, a slight boy who suffered from several bouts of childhood illness, had been the king of Spain from birth but he could not assume control of the country until he turned sixteen. Until then, his mother ruled in his stead. Aged just four, he spent some months in bed with what the newspapers described as an 'affliction of the heart'. It was rumoured that he might have hydrocephalus and crowds gathered at the palace gates every day for the latest news. Alphonso's patronage of Temple Street Hospital was gratefully appreciated and the sisters lost no time in drafting a letter to Madrid. They enclosed a picture donated by the sick children. In November 1897, the mother superior received the following reply:

My Dear Madam,

I had the honour to present to Her Majesty the Queen Regent of Spain the picture offered by you to His Majesty the King. Her Majesty was very grateful for your

Raffles had been held in support of the children's hospital since its early days in Buckingham Street. The home of Dr Thomas More Madden was often pressed into service as a ticket outlet for such events. (Hospital collection)

attention, and the picture will be placed in the 'Children's Refuge' of Maria Christina.

Your obedient servant,

Que besa su mano (who kisses your hand),

Luis Moreno[74]

In 1902, the young king put his childhood behind him for good when he acceded to the Spanish throne. The week of his majority was marked by great national festivities which included receptions, balls and bullfights. From the outset, France's *Le Figaro* described him as 'the happiest and best-loved of all the rulers of the earth'. A few years later, he went on to marry Princess Ina, who had visited Temple Street in 1900. It was thus by a strange coincidence that a girl who had once seen his portrait hanging in the front hall would herself become Queen Victoria Eugenie of Spain.

For the most part, however, it was the ordinary boys and girls of Ireland who made the guild a success. Moy Mell helped to keep the hospital open until the 1930s, when the Irish Sweepstakes began and still serves as a sweet reminder of how Ireland's young people can move mountains to help each other.

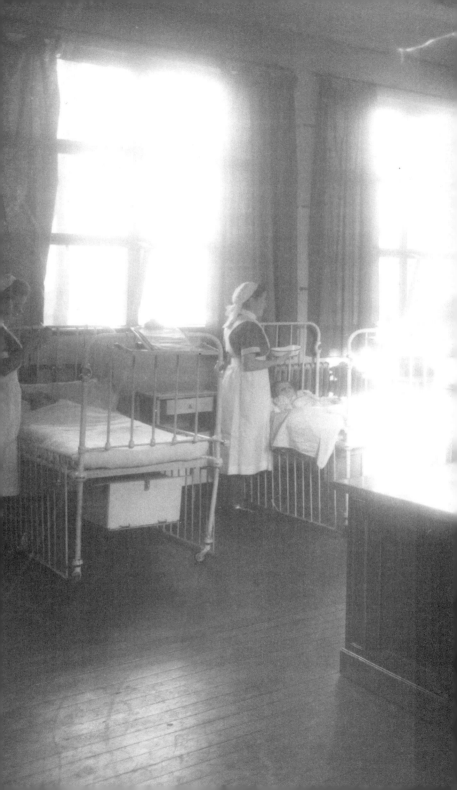

6
End of the
Victorian Era

Private ward at Temple Street, c.1930.
(Hospital collection)

round May 1899, a dispute arose at Temple Street when members of the medical staff raised concerns about how one of the nurses had been treated.[75] In response, Mother Superior Christina Hodgens wrote to Michael Staunton as head of the medical staff to ask that a number of the beds in each ward be devoted to eye and ear patients, adding that in the interest of expanding the hospital, greater adherence to administrative discipline was required. In particular, she reminded him of a rule, long since in abeyance, that each doctor needed to reapply for his post after serving a term of five years.[76] The doctors declined to accept this without discussion, however, as they felt that it would curtail their independence.

On 25 May 1899, Mr Staunton wrote to the mother superior. He outlined eight resolutions which, broadly speaking, aimed to put the power of making appointments into the hands of the doctors rather than the congregation and to appoint a lay board of managers 'to look after the interests of the sick children'.[77] This was similar to elsewhere in the British Isles, where lay people were beginning to occupy places on hospital boards and there was a growing consensus that hospital affairs, including the appointment of medical staff, ought not to be left solely in the hands of religious orders.[78] The mother superior put the matter before the archbishop of Dublin, however, and the hospital solicitor advised that it would be necessary to bring the doctors 'into line' by way of a settled agreement.[79] In her response dated 3 June, she was quick to remind Mr Staunton that:

The Sisters of Charity must continue to administer the internal working of the hospital for which they are and must be primarily responsible and arrange the respective duties of the sisterhood and the nursing staff by whom they are assisted according to the principles under which they have so long managed the hospital.[80]

In July 1899, Mr Staunton repeated the consultants' objection to the five-year rule. In response to this stance, the hospital solicitors advised that 'all the members of the staff hold their posts at the will of the Sisters of Charity', adding that the nuns were legal owners of the hospital with 'complete dominion over it'.[81] As a result, on 1 September 1899, Temple Street closed its doors to the public.

This did not attract as much attention as one might imagine. Victorian hospitals often closed for cleaning and disinfecting purposes or simply due to lack of funding.[82] This situation prevailed for the next two months – punctuated only by a response from the medical staff. 'The method of re-appointment which you suggest has been well described as a sword hung over our heads in case we become troublesome', they wrote on 5 September.[83] By 29 October, however, they sought to re-open negotiations by asking the mother superior to 'be good enough to inform the medical board when the hospital would reopen so that they might resume their work'.

Mr Staunton was the first to reapply for his hospital post. He must have cut quite a striking figure as he dismounted from his cab at Temple Street. He had lost a leg due to osteomyelitis and a contemporary newspaper photograph shows him wearing a top hat and frock coat. On arrival, he signed a simple form of acceptance based on an application form used by the Catholic University School of Medicine. Later, it was signed by most of the medical staff apart from Drs O'Carroll and Coleman, who decided to resign.[84] 'I am very glad indeed to know that the matter is so happily settled', the archbishop told Sr Hodgens on 8 November,

22 North Frederick Street,
Dublin.
Nov 8th 1899

Dear Mrs Hodgens,

I beg to apply for reappointment as Visiting Surgeon to the Children's Hosp. for a period of 5 years and remain

Yours Sincerely
M. C. Staunton
M.D. &c.

Letter from Mr Staunton to Mrs Hodgens dated 8 November 1899 in which the surgeon asks to be reappointed to Temple Street. (Hospital archive)

'I took it for granted all through that whatever happened, they would all stand or fall together'.[85]

That might have been an end to the matter, but on 13 January 1900 *The Lancet* decided to publish an article about the Temple Street affair.[86] Similar articles followed in the *Daily Independent* and *Evening Herald*. The archbishop advised Sr Hodgens not to respond. Instead, he quietly visited editorial offices across the city to ensure that there would be no further damaging articles. 'I found the directors of each very sympathetic', he reassured her, 'so that if we do our part tomorrow, there need be no fear of the result'.[87] Eventually, Dr Thomas More Madden, who had always stood firmly on the side of the sisters, wrote his own pamphlet in their defence. In his view, the sisters were responsible for making the hospital a success and had saved it from closing its doors in 1876. 'So much', he wrote, 'for the coup d'etat'.[88]

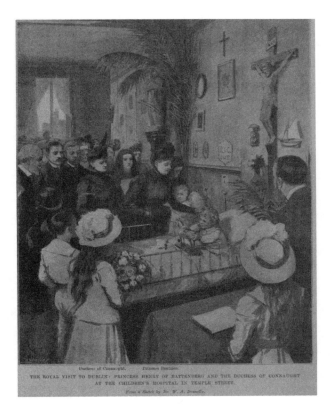

Royal visit to Temple Street as shown in the *Illustrated London News* of 21 April 1900. Depicted are the Duchess of Connaught, Prince Arthur of Connaught, Princess Margaret of Connaught, Princess Henry of Battenberg and her children, Princess Victoria Eugenie and Prince Leopold of Battenberg. On St. Agnes' Ward (Surgical Flat), they signed their names in the book of the Moy Mell Children's Guild. Soon afterwards, large visits like this were discontinued in the interest of the patients. (Courtesy of the British Library)

Today, this long forgotten dispute, though stressful enough for the hospital authorities at the time, is nevertheless an important part of Temple Street's history. It bore no reflection on the Sisters of Charity, who felt that they were acting in the best interests of their patients, or indeed the doctors, who expressed a similar duty of care. By April 1900, both sides of the house were able to present a united front when Queen Victoria's grandchildren, Prince Leopold and Princess Victoria Eugenie, visited. As they left flowers at each child's bedside, Temple Street was once again able to look to the future with optimism and hope.

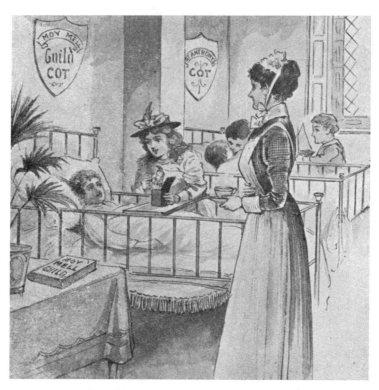

Cots were funded by voluntary contributions. The name of every benefactor was displayed on a heraldic shield at the head of each child's bed. Hospital annual report, 1897. (Temple Street archive)

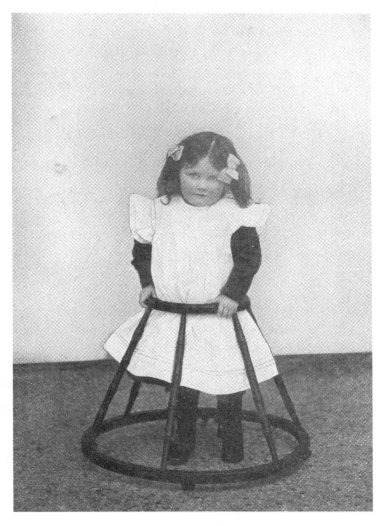

Child learning how to walk again after an operation.
(Temple Street Annual Report, 1914)

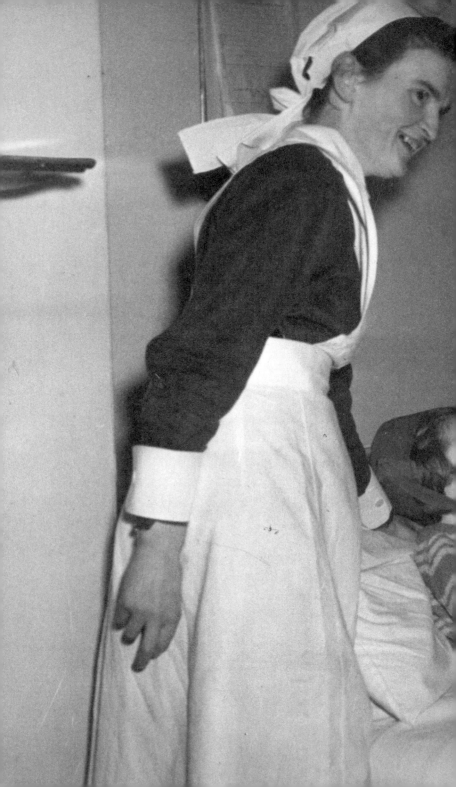

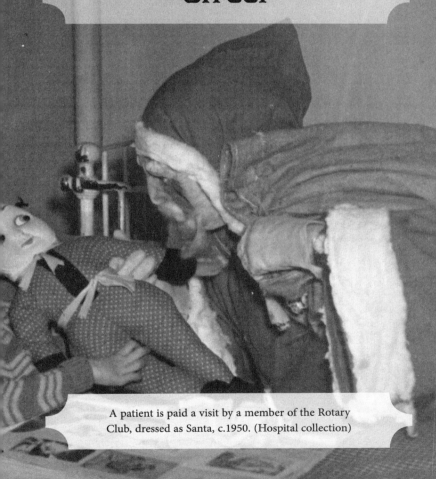

7
Christmas at Temple Street

A patient is paid a visit by a member of the Rotary
Club, dressed as Santa, c.1950. (Hospital collection)

Temple Street Children's Hospital

Temple Street Hospital has always occupied a special place in the hearts of Irish people, particularly in December when staff and visitors make special efforts to delight and entertain the patients. Every year, there is carol singing on the wards and on Christmas morning, the lord mayor attends Mass in the hospital chapel. These traditions began during the late Victorian period when the sisters, in an attempt to meet the heavy cost of running the hospital, opened their doors every year for a Christmas tree fête. 'Every ward was tastefully wreathed with holly and ivy', the *Freeman's Journal* of 29 December 1891 reported, 'and the walls were hung with bright pictures and coloured mottoes'.

The Christmas fête was usually held just prior to New Year and the centrepiece was a huge evergreen tree which occupied pride of place in one of the two large wards – an old drawing room that once formed part of the Earl of Bellomont's city mansion. As part of the preparations, the hospital's sixty or so inpatients were dressed in red flannel night jackets and each cot was decked out in white counterpanes and warm blankets. From early morning, they eagerly awaited the arrival of a throng of visitors – usually led by the wife of the lord lieutenant and her viceregal entourage and followed by the lord mayor, police commissioners and other dignitaries.

Fête day was very busy for Temple Street. Every year, upwards of 500 visitors gathered around the little cots and various entertainments were laid on for the patients. On 29 December 1893, the *Freeman's Journal* reported that:

> In the Convalescent Ward, a magic lantern entertainment was given by Mr Lawrence of O'Connell Street. All the scenes were of a humorous character, and it was a treat to hear the screams of delight with which they were received by the children.

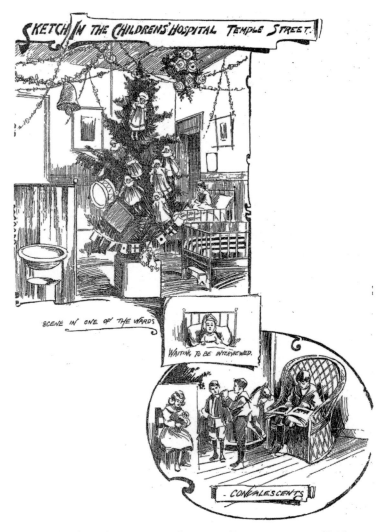

SKETCH IN THE CHILDRENS' HOSPITAL TEMPLE STREET.

SCENE IN ONE OF THE WARDS

WAITING TO BE INTERVIEWED.

CONVALESCENTS

Irish Independent, 29 December 1906. (Picture courtesy of Irish Newspaper Archive)

Many of the visitors handed out sixpence pieces, but the younger children had to be watched carefully since they were liable to eat them. Once the various dignitaries had visited all the wards, it was traditional for the lady lieutenant to distribute toys from the large Christmas tree. Some of the gifts were donated by wealthy patronesses such as the Marchioness of Derry, who included a card for each patient, the Royal Family at Windsor Castle, or by the German Empress Augusta of Saxe Weimar Eisenach, who was responsible for providing most of the toys in 1890 – rather poignantly, it seems, as she died on 7 January of that year.

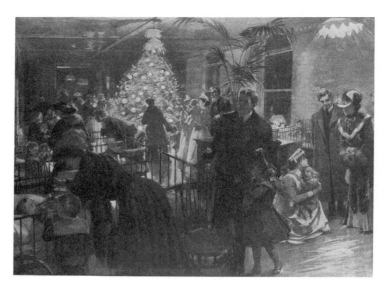

Visitors enjoy the Christmas tree fête, *Illustrated London* News, 31 December 1904. (Courtesy of the British Library)

Blissfully unaware of how great or small their visitors were, the children tucked into a meal of sweetmeats and fruit. Santa joined the festivities, but wore a green rather than a red costume. After the toys had been handed out, a concert was usually held around a piano in the largest of the halls. At the same time, tucked out of sight in the wooden dispensary, the sisters arranged a separate Christmas visit for the poor inner city children – an event that stood a world apart from the lavish parlour room spectacle:

> Last Tuesday, we invited a hundred of the real poor who had no dinner to get at home to a dinner party which comprised boiled mutton, bacon and cabbage and potatoes galore and to wind up, a huge plum pudding which had been boiled in an enamelled bucket. We all felt very happy although very tired when we saw the last of our poor little guests depart, each having received a nice toy, fruit and sweets to take home.[89]

In later years, the nuns decided that it would be better to give food to the local mothers so that they could cook their own Christmas dinner at home, but such charity was quite costly and only added to the hospital's seasonal expenses. The boilers were coal-fired as were the hearths in all the wards. Through their advertisements, the mother superior encouraged the public not to forget 'in the distribution of your Christmas Alms, the Hospital and Home for Sick Children'. The regional secretaries of the Moy Mell Children's Guild were similarly asked to send in 'warm hood capes for use in the garden' and 'combinations, cotton or woven'.[90]

Some Irish doctors felt that children would be better served by being catered for in special wards in the country's adult hospitals, particularly in the interest of avoiding cross infection, but shortly before Christmas 1885, Drs Thomas More Madden and J. McCullough told the Spenser Commission (which had been established to investigate hospital accommodation) that sick children deserved to be treated in a special environment of their own. Acting on their recommendation, Temple Street was allowed to continue its life-saving work and in 1890 it was certified by the Royal University of Ireland as a teaching hospital.[91] Thus, despite the odds, the fledging institution was able to remain open. In 1895, it received further assistance when the Countess Cadogan chose the Christmas fête as an ideal time to announce the commencement of a fundraising bazaar to be held in the Rotunda gardens every year.

In 1902, Dr More Madden died after sustaining an injury in a yachting accident. Because he had been so important to Temple Street in its formative years, his family decided to honour his memory by continuing a long-standing tradition. Each December, the smell of pine filled the front hall as a batch of fir trees, fresh from the family estate in Tinode, County Wicklow, were unloaded by horse-drawn cart. In 1912, these were decorated for the first time with festoons of garlanded electric light bulbs.

Christmas cards were another Edwardian novelty. In 1911, the Countess of Aberdeen sent eighty of them, one for each inpatient with an unusual crib design. By that time, the annual distribution of sixpences and sweetmeats of Victorian times had been replaced by an upsurge in gift-giving. Then, as now, it was the toys that evinced the most interest. 'A young fellow was weeping copiously', one visitor recalled. 'We later found him sitting in a chair by the fire, a smile on his little face. Poor little fellow! He had never seen so many toys before in his life.'[92]

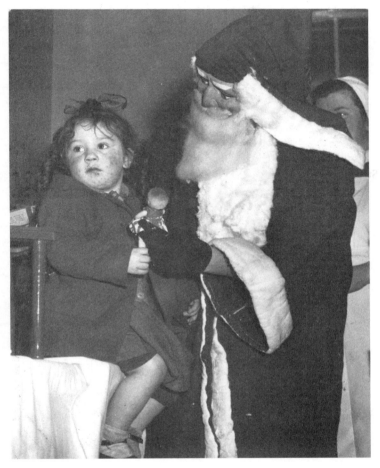

Sale of work at Temple Street, December 1961. (Hospital collection)

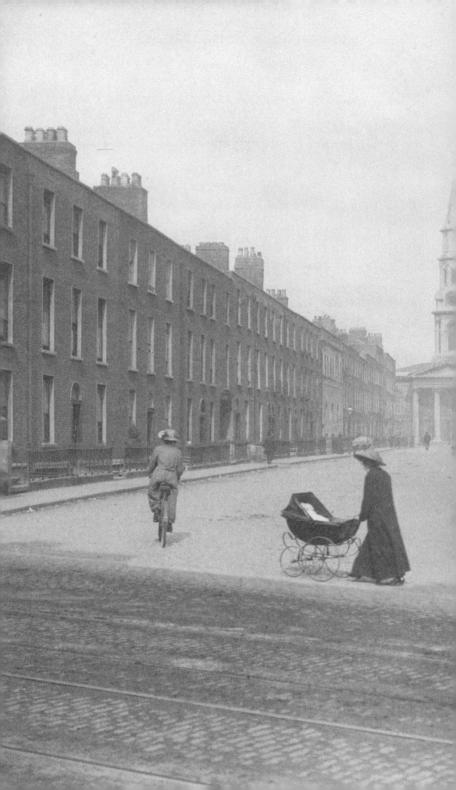

8
Children of the
Revolution (1916-1922)

Hardwicke Street. The newspaper stand suggests that the picture was taken after 1912. *The Daily News and Leader* only came on sale in that year. (Courtesy of National Library of Ireland)

The outbreak of the First World War affected Temple Street's revenues considerably.[93] The hospital still depended heavily on voluntary contributions, but with much-needed aid diverted to help the war effort, the sisters struggled to buy food, blankets, clothing and other essentials. By late 1914, Belgian refugees had begun to arrive via Red Cross ships and some of them needed medical care. Forty-six such vessels berthed in Dublin between October 1914 and February 1919.[94] On 6 November 1914, the Belgian Refugees Committee wrote to the medical commissioner of the Dublin County Borough to request that they 'supply medical assistance to Refugees in their area' and a number of the children came to Temple Street. Although details are scarce, it is probable that some of them belonged to the families who lodged in Great Denmark and Gardiner Streets.[95]

Other hospitals in the city were similarly burdened, in particular due to the number of doctors who had volunteered for army service overseas.[96] Later, a constant stream of casualties overwhelmed military medical facilities in France and Flanders and hospitals in Britain and Ireland were soon overrun. The authorities were unable to cope with the influx and civilian hospitals, hotels and other large buildings were pressed into service. In Dublin, these included the Richmond Hospital and the National Children's Hospital on Harcourt Street.

By the end of 1914, the wartime privation had become so severe at Temple Street that the Lady Superintendent, Miss O'Flynn, described it as having 'thrown an enormous burden on the resources of the hospital'. She was quick to remind the public that 'a large number of the children of our brave soldiers and sailors have been, and are being nursed back to health in the wards ... and a still larger number receive treatment in the Extern Department'.[97] Many of the hospital doctors also used the war to publicize the work that Temple Street was doing. At an annual fundraising meeting on 24 December 1915, Dr Boyd Barrett pointed out that more infants were dying in the tenements than soldiers on the battlefield and that, instead of helping sick children, it seemed to be 'more fashionable to make bandages and dressings for soldiers'. That year alone, he added, some 2,000 children of soldiers had attended for treatment.[98] The war also took its toll on staff morale. Many of the nuns had relatives fighting on the front and looked to the mother superior for consolation and support.[99] Little did they realise that, within a short time, war would arrive on their own doorstep.

Thus, on the eve of Easter Week 1916 – arguably the largest and most intense instance of a modern urban conflict in the British Isles until that point, Temple Street was not entirely removed from the realities of war.[100] At mid-day on Easter Monday 1916, some nurses rushed into the front hall. Their breathless cries that the 'Sinn Féiners have taken over the General Post Office' caused a flurry of excitement. That evening, the hospital received its first casualty, an eight-year-old called William Cullen who arrived by horse and cart. He was injured by a piece of stray glass when a rebel broke a window in nearby Findlater's shop on Sackville Street.[101] Over the following week, a total of eleven gunshot cases were admitted. Today, such a situation would call for instigation of the hospital's major disaster plan, but in 1916, the staff had to cope with the situation as best they could.

Early on Easter Monday, three companies of rebel volunteers (A, D and G) had been ordered to mobilise at St. George's Church adjacent to the hospital, from whence they were despatched to occupy the Mendicity Institute on Usher's Quay. Afterwards, rumours continued to abound in the city's newspapers that some soldiers had remained behind.[102] Con Colbert had used the National Theatre on Hardwicke Street to drill the Fianna in the days before Easter Week and, perhaps as a consequence of this, a barricade (one of the first to be erected that week) was thrown up at Findlater's Church at the top of Rutland Square.[103]

Many ordinary people were caught up in the conflict and children were particularly vulnerable. In January 1916, Seán Lemass accidentally shot his two-year-old brother Herbert as he was cleaning a firearm in their Capel Street home. At the inquest held in Temple Street Hospital, the jury remarked that 'something should be done to prevent young boys getting possession of firearms,' but no action was taken.[104] The Volunteers and Irish Citizen Army continued to prepare for

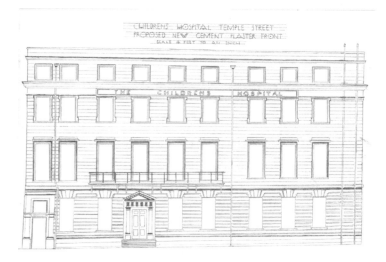

Like many other public buildings in Dublin, the frontage of Temple Street Hospital was damaged by gunfire during the revolutionary period. In 1931, Nos. 14 and 15 were unified with a grand new facade. This elevation is by William Henry Byrne & Son. (Picture courtesy of Irish Architectural Archive)

war and on the first day of the fighting, three children were killed, the youngest being John Francis Foster who was only two years old. He sustained a gunshot wound to the head on Church Street and died without medical assistance (although afterwards a priest took his body to the Richmond Hospital). The second was Christopher Cathcart, a ten-year-old boy from Charlemont Street who died at Portobello Barracks as a result of a 'gunshot wound'. The last was Patrick Fetherstone, from Long Lane off Dorset Street, a twelve-year-old boy who was injured by a bullet wound to the thigh. He died at Jervis Street Hospital from 'shock and haemorrhage'.[105]

At first, many of those who would later be admitted to Temple Street were taken to a dressing station set up by the Royal Army Medical Corps on nearby Dorset Street.[106] Others were taken to an emergency Red Cross Hospital situated in an empty house on North Great George's Street. On humanitarian grounds, staff there refused to comply with a British military directive to only admit their own personnel and later, Irish Parliamentary MP John Dillon would write that 'a steady stream of women, girls and young children have passed up this street'.[107]

In many instances, it was agreed that hospitals would be treated as neutral territory and that essential communication such as telephone lines should be left intact. In the case of Temple Street, however, visits to patients could only be obtained on the basis of a military permit and the hospital remained at constant risk from sniper fire. Of the thirteen doctors on its staff, only three lived nearby. The others were on the opposite side of the theatre of war and could not report for duty.[108] Some of these doctors certainly had experience treating gunshot wounds. They included surgeons Joseph Boyd Barrett, who had recently served with the Royal Army Medical Corps, and John

McArdle, a socialite who had operated on a bugler from the Royal Dublin Fusiliers when he was wounded in the leg by a Mauser.[109] Alongside these were sixteen live-in student nurses or 'probationers' who remained on hand to maintain essential services.[110]

On Tuesday, 25 April 1916, six beds were cleared in Temple Street's private ward – the first floor of an old Georgian House at No. 13 Upper Temple Street. It is not hard to understand why this part of the hospital was chosen. The house had been acquired during the 1890s and stood at a remove from the main wards, thus sparing other patients from witnessing the traumatic admission of adults and children. At the same time, it still allowed staff access to the kitchen, laundry and theatre without having to leave the safe confines of the hospital.

That same evening, a young man from Mullingar was admitted with a gunshot wound to the leg. 'He was a fine young fellow and was badly shot', one of the sisters recalled, 'he was got to bed but as he was bleeding badly, it was thought necessary to operate on him'.[111] Therein lay a dilemma, because the only doctor in the hospital was a house surgeon – a live-in student who, although unpaid, earned his 'assistant's fee' by helping consultant surgeons in the operating theatre.[112]

Since the anaesthetist was unavailable, one of the nuns had to act in his stead. At first, opiates appeared to relieve the young man's pain and the staff hoped he might recover, but a few days later, gangrene set in and his leg had to be amputated. Soldiers fighting on the front had already begun to treat their own wounds with antiseptic solutions such as iodine, carbolic acid and aluminium chloride, and while this would eventually become standard practice in Ireland, it was an innovation that came too late for some gunshot victims at Temple Street.[113]

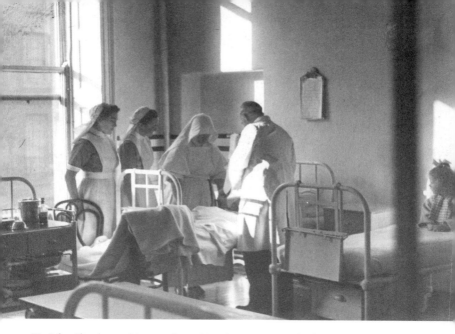

Dr John Shanley on his rounds, c.1930. As a young medical student, he witnessed the first shots of the 1916 Rising while returning from Mass in the Pro-Cathedral. Later, he performed an autopsy on the body of Irish Free State Commander, Michael Collins. During the 1940s, he became chairman of the Irish Red Cross society. (Hospital collection)

As Easter Week continued, doctors began to arrive via the adjacent laneways of Nerney's Court and Kelly's Row, which afforded some protection from the incessant gunfire. Not far from the hospital in Upper Dorset Street, the grocery and provision store belonging to Messrs McDonald Brothers had been relieved of several tons of bacon by looters and plate glass fragments lay all over the pavement. Many other shops on the street were completely stripped of their drapery, furniture, fruit and confectionary. The laneways around Hardwicke Street were subjected to a constant gunfire bombardment that battered the walls and smashed glass and woodwork into splinters.[114] Hardwicke Lane was particularly hard hit, with British Army gunfire damaging the windows, doors and locks of No. 5. Later, several of the residents claimed compensation for damage caused by 'military and looting'.[115]

One little girl who was sent out on a message not far from the hospital was killed as she returned to her home on nearby Wellington Street, but most of the casualties continued to stream in from thoroughfares that fringed the theatre of war – North King Street, Gloucester (Sean McDermott) Street, North Cumberland Street, Waterford Street and Parnell Street. On arrival, many of them were in a ragged and dirty condition and had to be cleaned before they could be treated properly. One such patient was Mary Kane, an adult patient from Waterford Street:

> On looking out of her window [she] received a bullet in the top of her skull. Her husband carried her on his back to Marlboro St Church, where she was anointed. As the haemorrhage was so profuse, a doctor arrested it, and stitched up the wound, on admission here. Next morning it had to be undone, as it was in a most septic state, owing to the filthy condition of the patient. She was able to return home in a week or two.[116]

As the fighting intensified, Temple Street Hospital received support from nearby Belvedere College and its rector, Father John Fahy. The sisters considered him to be 'a true friend' who was 'untiring in his efforts'. Nevertheless, he did not take chances and took great pains to keep priests and pupils off the streets during the fighting – something for which he was later praised by Ireland's interim military governor, General John Maxwell.[117] He and his fellow priests were granted permission to hear confessions and administer last sacraments but they 'came to attend the dying at the risk of their own lives'.[118] This was more than mere bluster on the part of the sisters:

> One night, Fr Fahy was hearing confessions. It was late when he was finished. Every time he opened the door to go home, he was fired at. Finally, through the influence of an army doctor whom he knew and who sent an ambulance to convey him to Belvedere, he made his way home.[119]

Supplies were now running low – particularly the beef tea and brandy upon which so many of the patients depended. Prior to the outbreak of hostilities, the sisters had received donations of fruit, vegetables and Easter eggs. Jacobs and Company (now held by the rebels) had even sent in 'cake and biscuits'.[120]

On Friday 28, Charles Kavanagh, a fifteen-year-old boy from North King Street, was admitted with a gunshot wound to the abdomen. He and his siblings had always been somewhat wayward and five years previously their father had been summoned to the police court for failing to keep them in school.[121] Although the circumstances of his shooting are unknown, the killing of over a dozen people in his locality by the South Staffordshire Regiment is well documented.

A doctor arrived by one of the lanes behind the hospital to perform abdominal surgery and, although no records of the procedure survive, contemporary *British Medical Journal* articles show how it might have been attempted. Everything depended on touch and observation but time was of the essence. To begin with, although Temple Street had a radiology department since 1907, it would have been difficult (although not impossible) to use X-rays to locate the bullet since the patient would have needed to remain still for a considerable length of time.[122] Instead, the abdomen was opened, packed with gauze to staunch the bleeding and the loops of intestine slowly disentangled and removed from the cavity. A single gunshot wound might result in numerous holes or tears as it traversed the abdomen – each of which needed to be sutured in turn with the attendant risk of contamination. In his description of an operation performed at Reigate and Redhill Hospital on a fifteen-year-old boy scout in 1917, Surgeon A.R. Walters gives the following account of the procedure: 'two mesenteric vessels were seen to be bleeding, and there were two perforations of the small intestine. The mesenteric vessels were tied'.[123] Not all cases were so routine, however. Edward Domville, who operated on a six-year-old boy who had been playing with a loaded rifle at the Royal Devon and Exeter Hospital in 1918, describes the scene that greeted him when he opened the abdomen:

> The lower part was found full of blood, which was wiped out and the pelvis packed with gauze; the coils of small intestine were then in turn taken out of the abdomen on to hot Cripps pads and the wounds in the small intestine sought for and in turn sutured; there were sixteen wounds, and from some of them portions of food and blood clot were protruding; the last hole was in the left mesocolon. The operation wound was sutured in layers and closed and the child put back to bed. [124]

A distinctive feature of this surgery was the use of methylated ether and a 'tincture of iodine' as an antiseptic measure – then quite novel but now standard when preparing a patient for theatre. Nevertheless, it was still extremely difficult to achieve surgical haemostasis and many children died on the operating table. Post-operatively, saline enemas with glucose were ordered every six hours and doctors watched for signs of a quickening pulse – a sure indication that something was amiss.

Unfortunately, the surgeon who operated on Charles Kavanagh was not successful and he joined the other deceased in a temporary mortuary. The bodies were wrapped in canvas or 'egg cases' which, considering the warm weather, would no doubt have created hygiene problems – a desperate situation that was replicated across the city. The Jesuits helped by travelling around the various hospitals to collect the bodies but when the man driving the horse and cart was shot dead, Fr Fahy had to take his place at the reins.

After a general surrender was called on Saturday, 29 April, it took some time for firing to cease in the Temple Street locality. Despite searches by the military on 1 May, continued sniping 'gave the military and the civil inhabitants a great deal of trouble.'[125] Information about the casualties treated at Temple Street was not released until the following month and respective accounts appeared in the *Irish Independent* and *Irish Times* of 17 May. After their 'awful week of strain and terror,' the sisters had to spend £811 on repairs to the hospital buildings – a sum which amounted to almost a quarter of the hospital's expenditure for the year.[126] Fundraising efforts were also disrupted for a number of months as they struggled to restore a normal service against the backdrop of a war-torn city.[127]

By the end of the Rising, civilian casualties vastly outnumbered those of the British army or rebels and it is estimated that at least 2,500 civilians were wounded.[128] Of these, 412 people died as a direct result of the fighting.[129] At the same time, almost 200 buildings lay in ruin in central Dublin with at least 100,000 people left homeless or in need of relief.[130] The City of Dublin Distress Committee donated 117 items of clothing to the sisters at Temple Street alone.[131]

Shortly afterwards, the sisters had to contend with an emergency of a different kind. Between 1918 and 1919, 20,057 Irish people were killed by Spanish Influenza according to official figures and a further 800,000 became ill. Globally, a staggering 40 to 100 million people were killed as the pandemic scourged the globe in three to four waves. Many of the children who contracted it lost their hair and it made their throats too sore to swallow food.[132] In October 1918, in the space of just twenty-four hours, twelve out of the eighteen domestic staff at Temple Street took sick, along with six nuns and a number of nurses. Those who were still on their feet tried to cope but it was obvious that the hospital had been stretched to breaking point:

> Those who were on their feet were tired to the utmost ... whole families were coming in. We were reduced to put babies in clothes baskets at the fire for no care was refused though where to put them was often a puzzle.

The community around Temple Street was particularly vulnerable because the disease affected two age groups in particular – children and young adults. Some people tried to treat themselves with hot towels, whiskey and quinine, and the nuns from Gardiner Street did their part by visiting families. They brought many of the children back to Temple Street and afterwards one of the nuns recalled: 'It was pitiful to see an old granny turning up as the sole survivor to rear the little orphans ... thank God we did not lose any of the sisters or the nurses although some of them were very bad with pneumonia and were anointed'.[133]

Around the same time, there was an upsurge in cases of tubercular bone disease – more common in children because the disease did not tend to settle in one place in the body as it did in adults. In order to isolate these patients from their healthier peers, some were removed to Cappagh in Finglas. Eventually, however, the number of cases necessitated the purchase of three huts from the American Naval Station at Cobh in Cork, two of which were used as wards with a third as a school.

In the middle of these preparations, the War of Independence broke out. 'The latter months of 1920 and beginning of 1921 were times of great strain on account of the disturbed state of the country', the sisters at Temple Street wrote. 'We were in constant dread of being raided by military from which no-one was safe. Many a night of terror we went through when their lorries full of drunken soldiers stopped outside.'[134] During the early hours of 14 November 1920, shots were heard near the hospital which woke many of the patients and frightened the nuns who tried to calm them. The following morning, several bullet marks were found on the front door and other parts of the building.

Black and Tans also raided local homes and businesses in their search for arms and, inevitably, children were caught up in the fighting. In January 1921, a lorry full of auxiliary officers knocked down a little girl on the North Circular Road, but they later called to Temple Street Hospital to see how she was doing.[135] Later that May, a baby was wounded by a bomb splinter when a Crossley Tender full of Royal Irish Constabulary officers was ambushed between King Street and Capel Street.[136] During one particular raid at 35 Hardwicke Street in September 1920, a woman informed the officer in charge that her young son was lying dead in Temple Street Hospital but 'even the schoolbag of the dead boy [was] examined'.[137] Joe O'Reilly, whose grandparents lived beside the hospital, recalls:

> My grandfather used to hide guns in No. 16 by pulling a brick out and putting them up the chimney and when my granny was younger, she used to bring the guns down to Father Mathew Hall from there disguised as a broom handle. When the curfew was on, he used to leave the door open so as people could sleep in the hallway. One time, when my grandmother's sister was pregnant, she tried to leave the house to help her but the Tans wouldn't let her; there was a British Army officer going by and he over-ruled the Black and Tans and escorted her down to her sisters' place. Because of that, the Tans came back the following night and ransacked the house but they never found any guns.[138]

In November 1920, a local newspaper man was almost killed on Temple Street by a volley of shots while he was on his rounds. Locals also sung a ballad about a homeless man who was shot in George's Pocket by the Black and Tans when he defiantly refused to put up his hands on the basis that he wouldn't do that for his own mother.[139]

Part of the reason why the sisters at Temple Street were under so much strain was because their mother superior, Polycarp Cummins, as well as the hospital matron, Margaret O'Flynn, had been actively aiding members of the IRA and ladies from Cumann na mBan.[140]

Children of the Revolution (1916-1922)

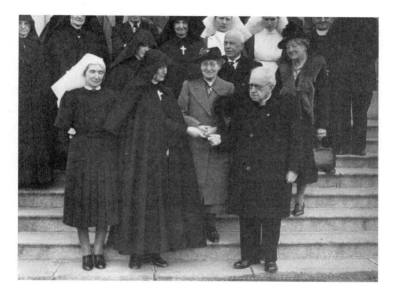

Rare photograph of Mother Polycarp Cummins with Archbishop William Walsh of Dublin, pictured shortly before his death in 1921. Both were supporters of the nationalist movement. (Hospital collection)

Mother Polycarp (meaning 'many fruits') had previously nursed at Temple Street but once she took charge of the community in 1913, she was soon sheltering 'young men, hardly more than boys'. Legend has it that she even helped Eamonn DeValera to disguise himself in a nun's habit out in Cappagh.[141] On one memorable occasion, Eilis Ui Chonaill and her colleagues from Cumann na mBan had to beat a hasty retreat through the rear of their Frederick Street premises carrying precious papers with them. A local publican guided them through the laneways to Temple Street Hospital, where 'Mother Polycarp received us with open arms and allowed us to deposit our files in a chest in the laboratory'.[142]

In 1920, Irish Republican Army revolutionary Cathal Brugha took refuge in the hospital boiler house, but on Bloody Sunday, a day of violence in Dublin during which thirty-one people were killed, the British Army was tipped off as to his whereabouts and plans were made to raid the premises. The operation began well before daybreak, culminating with the arrival of soldier-filled lorries at 8am. Fanning out, they searched not only the hospital but the nurses' home and the convent. The hospital was put under house arrest and the sisters were not allowed to have Mass.[143] Meanwhile, Brugha slipped out the back gate into a house owned by Mr Burke, the hospital boiler man who already had a history of harbouring fugitives.[144] When Burke arrived home for his lunch, he found the rebel sitting at his kitchen table with two revolvers in his hands. Brugha's brother Alfred describes the conversation that ensued:

> Burke asked him did he know the place was surrounded. Cathal said he did, and he would advise him, if possible to get the family away ... He appealed to Cathal to go into the house, but Cathal remained there, and passed the remark, 'If those people come in, you will find my dead body there' pointing to the place 'and don't be surprised to find six or seven of the bodies of our visitors!'[145]

Later, the boiler man and his son were taken away for questioning but the army met its match in the stern figure of Mother Polycarp, who saw to it that Brugha was able to make his escape. In return for such assistance, the IRA and Cumann na mBan seized a consignment of boot and floor polish, matches and household articles from British-friendly shops which they 'handed over mostly to Temple St. Hospital, which was very glad to receive them'.[146]

Children of the Revolution (1916-1922)

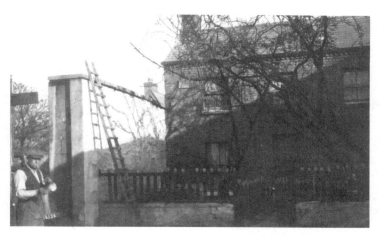

Back gate of Temple Street Hospital adjacent to Home Cottage, St Anthony's Place on 11 November 1937 at noon. It was through this entrance that members of Cumann na mBan entrusted weapons and documents to the safekeeping of Mother Polycarp. (Hospital collection)

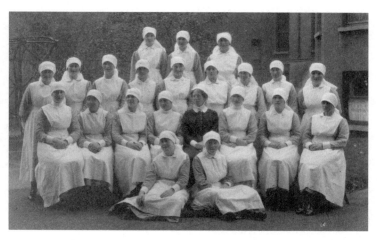

Born in 1864, Margaret O'Flynn from Elphin, County Roscommon (pictured here in the dark dress near the centre) was matron of Temple Street Hospital until the late 1920s. Before training as a nurse, she worked as a school monitor. Out of her own money, she bought bales of cotton which she gave to the students so that they could make underwear and other garments. Her sister, also a nurse, married a surgeon in Bombay, India and one of her brothers also worked in the Indian secret service. During the War of Independence, she actively aided members of the IRA and Cumann na mBan. (Hospital collection)

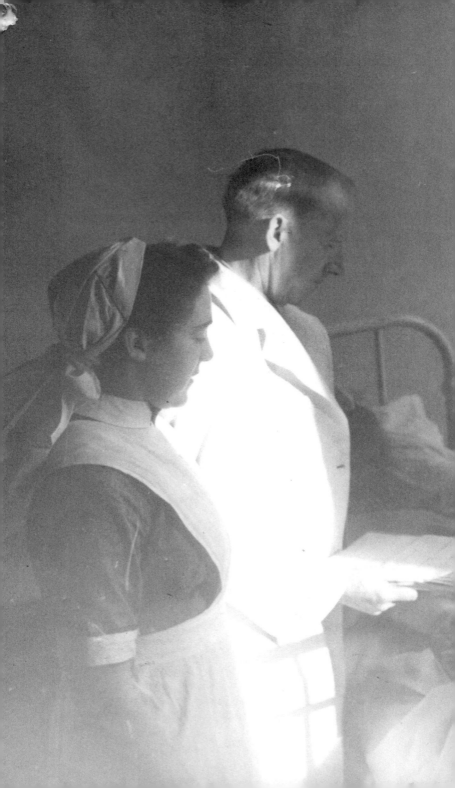

9
The Emergency Years
(1939-1945)

Dr John Shanley on his ward round, 1930s.
(Hospital collection)

During the 1940s, Temple Street Hospital continued to benefit from medical advances. Antibiotics such as penicillin were beginning to win the war against infection and better developed anaesthetic techniques, coupled with endotracheal intubation, were making surgical procedures safer. Nevertheless, there was no immunisation against bacterial infections such as diphtheria and it was a common sight to see shivering, red-blanketed nurses being removed from Temple Street to Cork Street Fever Hospital.

The Second World War (known euphemistically in Ireland as 'the Emergency') brought its own challenges. As soon as hostilities began in 1939, the superioress, Mother Camillus O'Donoghue, began to stockpile food and clothing, which included necessaries such as drugs, chemicals, dressings, X-ray films, soap and coal. On 12 October 1940, she saw to it that the following notice was displayed in public areas, including the hospital's brand-new A&E department:

> It should not be necessary to remind hospitals that the gravity of the present emergency situation demands that the strictest measure of economy, consistent with efficient services, should be enforced in every sphere of hospital work.[147]

In short order, the hospital garden was turned into an allotment for growing potatoes and cabbages. Occasionally, the more daring medical students raided it at night for rhubarb, which they used to make tarts. At the same time, cement bomb shelters were erected outside in Temple Street as well as in the hospital grounds by the authorities.

THE CHILDREN'S HOSPITAL,

TELEPHONE 45314.

TEMPLE STREET, NORTH.
DUBLIN. C.14.

N O T I C E

(Extract from letter received from Hospitals Commission on
12th October 1940)

"It should not be necessary to remind hospitals that the
gravity of the present emergency situation demands that the
strictest measure of economy, consistent with efficient
services, should be enforced in every sphere of hospital work.
Hospitals are again referred to the circular letter dated
12th August 1940 issued to them by the Minister for Local
Government and Public Health, and particularly to the annexed
copy of the Commission's report in which it was recommended
that hospitals should be warned:-

(1) To economise and avoid wastefulness in the use of food,
fuel, linen and domestic items generally.

(2) To economise in the use of medicines which may prove
irreplaceable and which may be urgently needed in
time of national emergency.

(3) To avoid increases in staff and personnel which would
involve increases in working expenses.

(4) To confine expenditure on maintenance of buildings to
items of absolute necessity and to consult the
Minister or the Commission whenever items involving
large outlay are in contemplation.

(5) To ensure that the greatest care is taken of existing
equipment, both medical and mechanical, as replacement
may not be possible."

In view of the above I would be glad of the co-operation
of the staff in effecting economy wherever possible.

SUPERIOR.

This notice, which dates from 18 October 1940, was placed in all
prominent parts of the hospital. It cautioned staff to economise and
avoid wastefulness – a policy that was maintained for the duration of the
Emergency. (Hospital collection)

In total, the hospital paid £684.4.6 on air-raid precautions; after the
war it was able to recoup some of this money from Dublin Corporation
and the Department of Defence.[148] Coal was also rationed along with
many other commodities and a journey to Dublin by train became an
ordeal for patients who lived further afield. Niall Durney (seventy-one)
from Waterford sustained bad burns when a stone hot water bottle

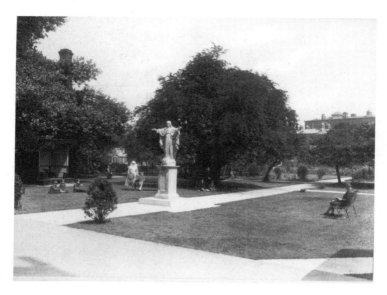

During the Emergency, the hospital garden was turned over to the planting of vegetables. (Hospital collection)

leaked in his bed and he had to be taken to Temple Street for regular check-ups. 'The train used to take about five and a half hours to get to Dublin', he recalls. 'Sure the engines were all running on turf then; there was nothing else and you'd see it all along the track.'[149]

The hospital was also affected by the war in other, more direct ways. In 1939, Dr John Shanley, who claimed to be Ireland's first full-time paediatric surgeon, co-founded the Irish Red Cross. In April 1941, he sent a number of Temple Street nurses to assist the society's efforts to help Northern Irish refugees who had been made homeless by bombing raids.[150]

When retired hospital porter Gerry Dudley started work at the hospital in 1945, the windows along the A&E laneway still had sandbags in them.[151] Fortunately, these were never needed, although the North Strand bombings on the night of 31 May 1941 did cause some damage – a reminder to staff and patients that the war was not far away. Bridget Dempsey (ninety-two), then a member of the household staff, recalls:

> I remember the night of the bombing. We were in bed at about two o'clock in the morning when the planes crossed over. If the bomb had of dropped five minutes before, we'd have had it because it would have fell in the hospital garden. Mr Hawes, the hall porter, was coming down the steps to look out; he got a bang on the back of the hand from a stone and his hand was out for a long time. That night, we were put to working in Casualty. They all came in – we had to help on the wards with the beds and we looked after the families and fed them.[152]

At the same time, the hospital needed to sustain its programme of expansion to cater for new services and its catchment area continued to grow. In August 1932, the mother superior travelled to the Continent to learn how a modern hospital ought to be run. Around the same time, Fraulein Mia Rotter arrived from Professor Moll's famous clinic in Vienna to set up a new dietetic department.[153] That same year, St. Patrick's baby ward was opened. During the summer, the little infants sitting up in their cots with their green adjustable cot shades was one of the most heart-warming sights in the hospital. The following year, the Irish Hospitals' Commissions recommended that fifty additional beds be installed in order to alleviate overcrowding (in some cases, there was more than one child to a bed) and to prevent sick children from being sent home at a point too early in their convalescence.[154] By the start of the war, the sisters had also sought to develop a new isolation block and to develop a house on the grounds for housing its domestic staff. Many of the children who were admitted had rheumatic fever, which was considered to be highly contagious and they had to be kept apart.

Such care was expensive, however. Since March 1931, the hospital had been in receipt of money from the newly established Irish Hospital Sweepstakes fund, but this was curtailed by the government on the basis that the sisters earned money from their shares in various Irish railways and banks as well as the Irish Sugar Company and Guinness. With the outbreak of hostilities, however, almost all of the hospital's stocks and shares dropped sharply in value and some even became 'unsaleable'.[155] In addition, Dublin Corporation halved its annual grant of £400. The government also alleged that Temple Street earned money from St. Anthony's shrine – a claim that the hospital auditors and accountants were quick to dismiss: 'Subscriptions and donations … were sent by the greater proportion of the donors with the request that they be used for St. Anthony's Bread [which] meant the distribution in one form or another to the poor and needy'.[156] Many local people had come to depend heavily on the hospital for support and the sister almoner distributed an average of forty food tickets per day – a figure that remained constant into the 1950s. The nuns visited approximately 300 homes a year, providing clothing and other essentials and they sent some of the children on a holiday to Baldoyle. Finances were further strained when Nos. 13 and 14 Hardwicke Place, which the hospital had acquired in order to enlarge the site, proved unsafe and had to be demolished along with 35 George's Place. Likewise, Nos. 16 and 17 Temple Street, which it purchased in 1938 under a compulsory purchase order, could not be renovated due to lack of funds.[157]

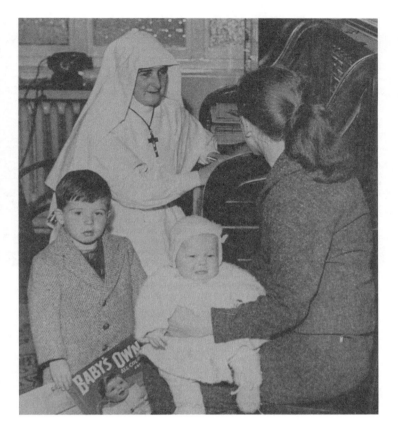

Hospital almoner, Sr. Frances Regis at work, c.1960. Her department dispensed meal tickets – a forerunner of today's social work service. (Hospital collection)

Fortunately, the hospital authorities were able to make a persuasive argument for developing badly needed new facilities. The new isolation block known as St. Michael's finally opened in 1940 and its babies, particularly those who had broncho-pneumonia, benefitted from new drugs such as sulphonamide and sulfapyradine, which reduced the mortality rate to as low as six percent – something that my infant father, born in March

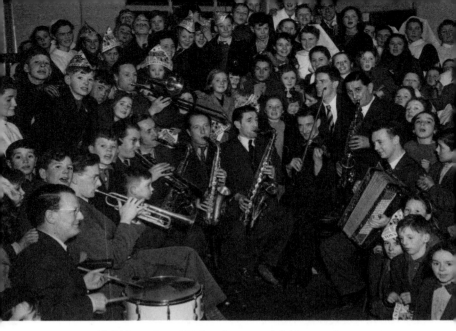

Phil Murtagh and his band entertain children in the outpatient department, December 1944. This part of the hospital is still used for TV3's annual Christmas broadcast. (Hospital collection)

of that year, benefited directly from.[158] When he was admitted to St. Michael's for a two-week inpatient stay in December 1940, he was one of the first children not to undergo the old regimen – generous use of oxygen and brandy.

By 1944, the war had become so serious that none of the sisters who were living in Dublin went home to the country at Christmas. Nevertheless, staff kept up morale, as William Sheridan (eighty-nine) from St. Anthony's Place recalls:

> I remember there was a bit of a do in the hospital for Vera Lynn, the English singer who sang 'We'll Meet Again' for the troops during the war. I remember her being a big tall woman and there was a maypole that we all danced around.[159]

The Emergency Years (1939-1945)

In December 1944, a musician attached to Phil Murtagh's band was so grateful for the care that his sick child had been given that he arranged for the band to play free of charge. The sisters struggled to man the doors as almost 200 children flooded into the outpatient department where tables had been piled high with tea, cakes, fruit and sweets.

By the end of the war the following May, the air raid shelters were removed from the hospital grounds and the new mortuary, which had been used as a bomb shelter since 1939, was restored to its original purpose. Soon afterwards, new hospital employees, some from Eastern Europe, arrived with their own stories to tell about the horrors of war. Among them was Ukrainian laundry worker Anna Guschkowska, who was met on her arrival in Dublin by the sisters. 'We have much to be grateful for', one nun wrote. 'Our country remained neutral; we were preserved from numerous dangers of every sort.'[160]

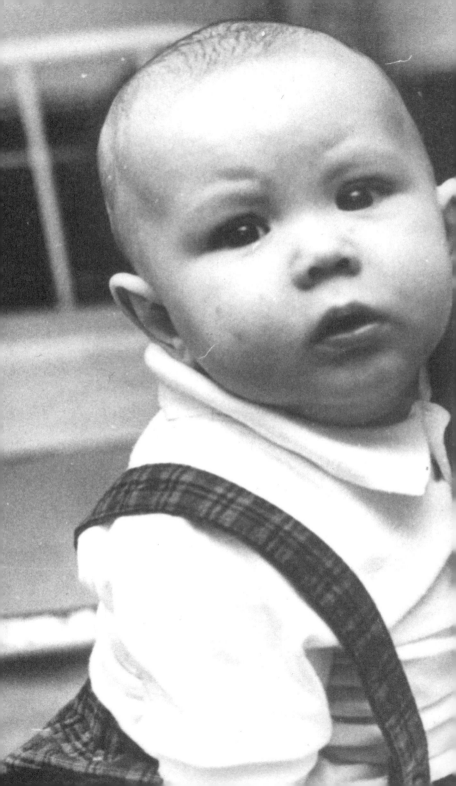

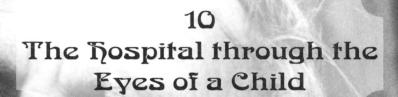

10
The Hospital through the Eyes of a Child

Head porter Paddy Doyle with Daniel Hughes from the
Ashbourne Road, County Dublin. Paddy, whose name
was synonymous with Temple Street, started work there in 1941.
(Hospital collection)

Temple Street Children's Hospital

Those children who attend hospital today have a far different experience than their counterparts half a century ago. Thanks to charitable organisations like *Youbyou*, their emotional needs are met on a daily basis through arts and crafts, multi-sensory areas, formal school programmes and interaction with play specialists. Every attempt is made to normalise the inpatient experience – in short, to make the hospital a home away from home.

Prior to the 1970s, however, the reality was much different. In most cases families could not visit and the pavement outside was often thronged with parents who stood back from the railings to wave up at little faces pressed against the window panes. Antoinette Murray (sixty-eight) who was admitted to Temple Street in the late 1950s after she was knocked down by a bus near Walton's music shop, recalls: 'I couldn't have complained over food or treatment; the only thing I missed was that my parents could only get in on Saturday or Sunday; my uncle used to come if my mother wasn't able. I'd see his hat down below at the front door and know that he was waiting for me. He used to bring in MiWadi and I'd have that diluted for the week.'[161] Additional allowances were made for more critically ill children. Rita O'Keeffe (née: Cunningham), who contracted meningitis, remembers that things were touch and go: 'Every morning, my dad, before he went to work, would spend one hour with me and again at lunch time. He went home every evening to let my mam up to visit me as he had to mind my sister and brother. That went on for over four and a half years.'[162]

For parents, the experience was often traumatic and not something to be spoken about lightly. Maureen Cunningham (seventy-seven), who underwent a bowel operation in 1938 when she was just four and a half months old, recalls:

My mother did say there was something in the *Mail* about it but she was a quiet woman. I remember her and my granny sometimes saying 'you're a grand little miracle' but she didn't like to dwell on the past; she lost two other children after me; she used to say to me, 'I nearly lost you as well'.[163]

In retrospect, many of the children also felt that their time at the hospital was little short of miraculous. When Declan Dunne from Timolin, County Wicklow took ill as a baby in 1959, he was rushed immediately to Temple Street:

Me father had a new Volkswagen Beetle. In those days the roads were very bad and he put sparks into them. He wasn't going to stop anyhow. He was a big strong man that done an awful lot of heavy work in his youth; he would walk through a locked door but he was a very bad patient. They done an operation where they split all me fingers and toes to try and drain the poison out of the bloodstream; they told me mother and father that as far as they were concerned there was no hope. The news that they got was that I was after dying. I don't know what fancy instruments they had but then I started up again. I had died for five minutes but the body had come back. That was a great story with my mother and father all through my childhood years.[164]

Others hold memories from a time when they were very young, when their language skills were not so well developed or when they were feverish, drifting in and out of consciousness. It is no wonder, then, that sometimes strange associations of colour and sound were preserved. Audrey Nicholson (eighty-five) remembers that she spent some time at Temple Street in 1929 when she was one and a half years old with peritonitis:

> When my mother went in to have a look at me they had a white screen around the cot. She was told that if I could keep down a spoonful of water, I would live. My appendix had burst but because mum had never given me any meat to eat, there was no poison. We were right beside St. George's Church. 'Those bloody bells', mum used to say, because they kept me awake. Do you want to want to know a funny thing about the white screen? Until I was confirmed in the same church, every time I heard the bells, I used to get a white mist in front of my eyes.[165]

Until the late 1980s, the transport network was not as well developed as it is today and many of the children who came from outside Dublin received no visitors. As a result, the staff developed close bonds with their little charges – particularly those who were in for a long-term stay. Some of the nurses were even allowed to take them home at weekends. Those attachments could sometimes be problematic, however, as Helen Connell, whose brother spent some time at Temple Street in 1964, attests: 'He used to get so upset when we came to visit. He was after kind of getting used to the nurses and it nearly made him worse to see us. We used to just stand there looking through a slit in the door'. At just thirteen years old, Helen felt helpless so she paid a visit to the home of Dicky Rock and asked him to play a charity concert at the hospital. She will

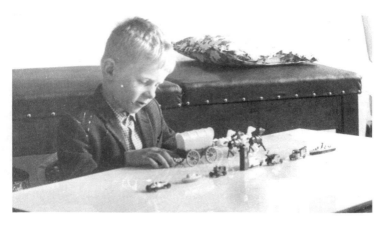

Boy plays with a cowboy and Indian set, c.1960. Some other toys are lined up alongside. (Hospital collection)

always remember him singing 'Every Step of the Way' with her brother standing on stage.[166]

A large number of children were admitted with chest conditions – a common result of damp, foggy conditions in the city's tenements. Among them was the author Brendan Behan, who took ill after standing at a rainy football match in Croke Park on 23 September 1934:

> I could have changed my clothes and got into bed only half Ireland seemed to have got themselves into our street, looking for shelter ... in our house we had a hooley, and the measure of our accommodation was not such that we could have a hooley and get into bed at the same time. My father played the fiddle, amiable as always, anything from 'The Blackbird' to 'The Lady in Red' and we danced and sang the night away, till in very short order I got pneumonia and found myself in Temple Street Children's Hospital.[167]

Some injuries were specific to a particular time and place. During the 1940s and '50s, many children caught and injured their heels in the spokes of bicycle wheels as a consequence of sitting on the carrier or crossbar. The 'maul' was a popular game in Dublin which involved playing with manhole covers or 'shores' and fractures caused as a result of trying to retrieve marbles from them were common. Those with orthopaedic problems like Perthe's disease or congenital dislocated hips spent a long time in bed with their legs suspended in the cot with a wooden block to keep them in position. John O'Sullivan (seventy-seven) from Raynestown in County Meath recalls spending two months lying supine after he was kicked by a pony in the face. 'I had to have my two arms tied up with cardboard so as they couldn't

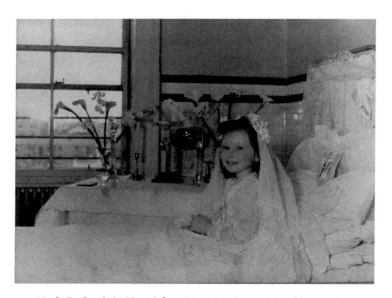

Nuala Fischer (née: Harris) from Mountjoy Street pictured here on her Communion day in 1944. Nuala was admitted to Temple Street with pneumonia, pleurisy and rheumatic fever. She was so ill that she had to be isolated. On the day this picture was taken, the children on the ward received a welcome treat from Mr Vella's ice-cream parlour. (Courtesy of Nuala Fischer)

bend. There used to be a glass house on the roof and on a fine day, they'd push the beds out for a bit of fresh air'.[168] Likewise, Bernie Kenna from Donnycarney, who spent three years recovering from bad burns, spent most of her time in bed with a cage over it. During those years, most if not all of the wards were managed by nuns who were also trained nurses. 'A lovely nun used to pray at me bed every night and she had a picture of Our Lady that used to shine and sing a song', she recalls. 'She bought me my communion dress but I had to be carried up to the altar. Years after, I visited the hospital when my youngest sister was knocked down. The same nun was still there. She came over and just put her arms around me. She was so delighted to see me. "I didn't think you would grow an inch", she said. "You're lovely", she kept saying, "You're lovely".[169]

Besides their treatment, the children were naturally curious about the work that went on in the ward. Antoinette Murray remembers that the nurses kept everything spotless: 'They didn't leave a spot of dust and at mealtimes we all had to wear a bib so as not to dirty our jammies. They used to clean the beds down to the rubber'.[170] Michael Foran, who was admitted for appendicitis in 1960, has a similar recollection:

The hospital was like the engine room of a ship – all pipes and it was part of the nurses' job to be down cleaning them and all along the bottom of the walls. Afterwards, the nuns would come along with their white gloves and run a finger along that way to check for dust.[171]

The public patients were served a meal from the ward kitchen but the food was very basic. Tea was boiled up in a single flask with the milk and sugar mixed together. 'The main thing I remember is the taste and smell of lukewarm tea from a plastic cup', Tom Burnell writes. 'Yeuch!'[172] In Top Flat Ward, Sr Arsenius knew all of the patients by ailment. When the dinner trolley arrived she used to tell the nurses, 'Give that to the eye'; 'Give that to the leg'. She kept everything in good order but on one occasion, a Greek surgical registrar incurred her wrath. Blessed with a charming manner and disarming smile, he took her face in both hands and exclaimed: 'Sister, when you are angry, I just love you!'[173] In the private areas, the experience was slightly different. There, the patients were treated to a silver service – little milk jugs, a separate sugar bowl and more fuss. On St. Philomena's Ward, Sr Catherine Aquinas could be heard phoning parents to put them at their ease. 'Oh yes, he's fine. He's had two spoonfuls of rice today'.

As a treat, many of the convalescent children were taken down to the forge by hospital porter Paddy Doyle. Rita O'Keeffe has a similar memory: 'The doctor used to wheel my bed over to the window to watch the men shoe the horses. They used to wave up at me as they did their work'.[174]

At the same time, Temple Street was also important to generations of local children, many of whom piled into the A&E department with their friends in tow. At dinner hour, it was not uncommon for a mother to ask, 'Who put them stitches in for you?' Lorraine Robertson (née Sheridan) from Hardwicke Street flats recalls:

We used to scut on the buses which had a bar on the back of them. In those days, they turned off Dorset Street into Hardwicke Street. We used to jump on at the top of the road and hold the bar until it got to Frederick Street and the conductor got on. If anything happened to us, me ma would send us over to Temple Street. 'Run over and

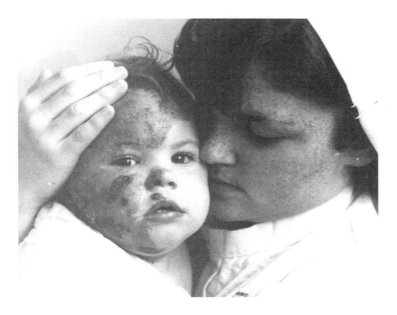

Joanna Kerins, aged 13 months, pictured here in the hospital burns unit on 11 November 1979. Hospital life could be particularly difficult for such children but a cuddle made all the difference. (Hospital collection).

get a plaster', she'd say. Our parents never brought us to hospital and you'd end up going in with maybe four or five of your friends. Paddy Doyle was the porter on the desk and he used to have a big box of them. He was a very friendly man and all the kids loved him.[175]

Inevitably, as retired nurse Eileen McLoughlin attests, the A&E staff were on the receiving end of all this activity:

It got a little bit busier in the summer because you had children falling off the backs of trucks. I remember on my first day hearing a new word – 'I'm after been scutting miss'. At that time, there would be a lot of local children.

When I was on night duty, we had great cooperation from the Dublin Fire Brigade Paramedics (DFB) but there were occasions when we had to remind them that there was no point in bringing in a child or a baby from their home environment and not being able to give any history.[176]

Towards the end of the 1950s, the old Georgian houses in Hardwicke Street and George's Pocket became vast, dilapidated playgrounds where children could be found crossing exposed joists and chasing each other through the crumbling yards and hallways. Brian Browning from Hardwicke Street Flats recalls: 'When the old houses were being knocked down and the flats were being built, I was being chased by another fella when I met a railing at a 45 degree angle; it was low enough to hit me and it bust me eye'.[177]

More recently, this author was walking towards Mountjoy Square one summer's evening when he came across a group of children standing around a boy on Gardiner Row. A discarded flicker scooter told its own story. 'I think he's after breaking his leg mister', a girl explained. 'Here, are you a doctor?' another said. Soon, a diminutive nurse appeared from the archway of Nerney's Court pushing a wheelchair. When she reached the group, she asked them to move back and give the lad some air. Within a few minutes, she was pushing him back towards A&E – his curious friends in tow.

During the early 1970s, the medical community took a closer interest in hospital life from a child's perspective. It was no longer acceptable to treat patients like miniature adults at best or at worst, infants who should be seen and not heard. In May 1970, the *British Medical Journal* voiced an emerging consensus – that as far as possible, hospitals ought to be made less intimidating places for sick children. In his address to the annual scientific meeting of the Irish Paediatric Association in Temple Street Hospital, the Minister for Health, Mr Childers expanded on the theme. Sick children were 'in greatest need of the security of familiar faces and surroundings'.[178]

But the hospital had already taken the lead – a quiet revolution in paediatric healthcare was underway. In 1968, the hospital school opened its doors for the first time and from the outset, its teachers quickly realised that they were in a somewhat unique situation. They constantly needed to adapt to the educational requirements of a diverse group of patients while at the same time providing a sense of normality in an otherwise uncertain environment. Ex-principal Ms Phil Dawson perhaps summed it up best when she recalled the words of the *sean-fhocal*: "*Mol an Óige agus tiocfaidh siad*".

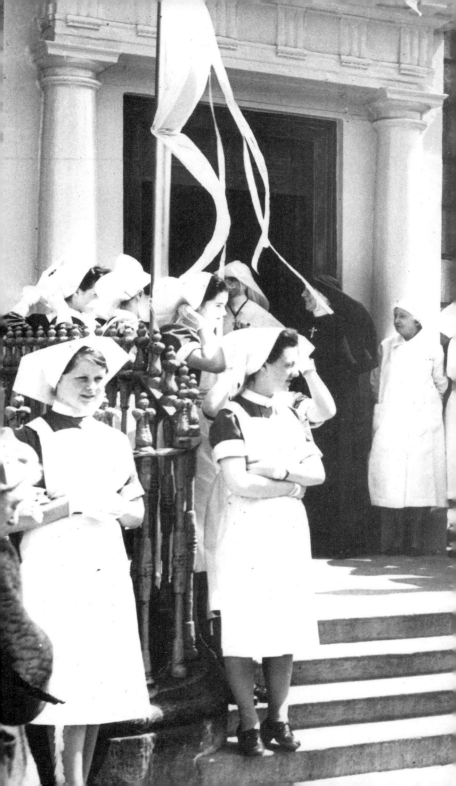

11
Children's Nursing

Nurses led by Matron May Hughes prepare for the
visit of Dr Fulton Sheen, an American Roman Catholic
Bishop and pioneer of television evangelism who was in Ireland
for the Patrician Congress of 1961. (Hospital collection)

In the early days, it was common for the porters at Temple Street to assist in bandaging a patient's wounds or, in the absence of modern anaesthesia, attend a surgeon at an operation. As the hospital began to expand, however, it soon became apparent that additional help was required. During the 1880s, the mother superior placed an advertisement for nurses. Each candidate needed to be under twenty-five years of age (or over if she was willing to part with one guinea per week) and the entrance fee was £10. Before attending an interview, she needed to provide written testimonials of good character and afterwards to provide two uniform dresses, six aprons and two caps. If she lasted her first three months, an indoor uniform was supplied.

The hospital nursing records from 1917 to 1939 reveal a lot about the composition of probationers at Temple Street. Of the 299 candidates, some two-thirds came from outside the city and of those almost half had a farm upbringing. The addresses and paternal professions of the remaining third from Dublin puts them in an almost exclusively upper middle-class category – the largest number of admissions coming from the townships of Clontarf, Drumcondra and Rathmines.[179] By and large, the girls were extremely young – some just sixteen years old – and as late as the 1950s, training was extremely hands on. On arrival, they were expected to start work immediately and pick up skills as they went along, as Teresa O'Connell (née Collins) explains:

I remember going to Stanhope Street to the nuns for my uniform which I had to pay for. You went into your bedroom the first night and the next one, you were on duty. We were told to bring cases with us but Maureen McGuinness and I thought that they were for books.

The two of us arrived onto Top Flat thinking that we were there to study. We put the cases straight into Sr Arsenius's press. 'Who owns these?' she shouted. She poked them out and got us to bring them right back to our room. There was no studying first – we were there to work.[180]

During their first year at Temple Street, student nurses attended lectures but there was no special treatment for those who had been on night duty. 'You just stayed up and went down to the lecture room', Collette Delaney recalls. 'Classes lasted until 11am and it might be three weeks before you got a night off. It was hard but we didn't know any better'.[181] In the early days, lectures were delivered by the hospital doctors or lady superintendent and since infectious cases were not admitted, probationers were sent on a special course to Cork Street Fever Hospital. They could not fully qualify until they put in some time at a general hospital however. Exams were held at intervals and when not on active duty, they were expected to undertake needlework or household chores. They were not allowed to take money from patients or friends under any circumstances and were liable for instant dismissal for any act of 'moral delinquency'.

In the meantime, the lady superintendent charted the career of each student in scrupulous detail. The high expectation held by the parents of rural girls is evident from the registers as is the strictness enforced in matters of appearance and hygiene. The superintendent frowned upon an unhealthy interest in 'outside pleasures' but this had little effect on some girls who got married during their summer holidays and never came back. Besides the

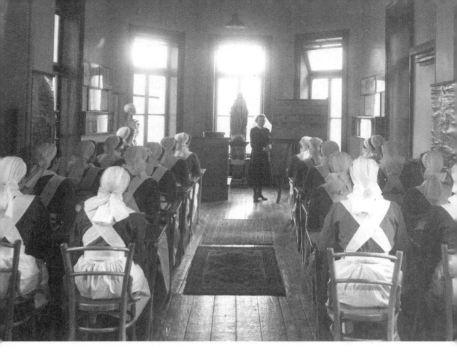

Nurse tutor, Ms Hughes at work. By the 1930s, approximately thirty probationers enrolled every year. They followed a General Nursing Council syllabus that replaced subjects such as cookery. Students were expected to learn anatomy, physiology, hygiene and bacteriology. (Hospital collection)

constructive comments, the registers also contain less favourable remarks such as: 'An intelligent capable girl who ought to make a good nurse but was evidently spoilt in upbringing and sulked like a bold child when corrected for faults'. For the most, part however, the general impression is that the young ladies were held in high regard.

In the early days, nurses took their breakfast at 6.35am after which the household servants sat down for their own meal, followed by the lady superintendent, staff nurses and medical staff. At the turn of the twentieth century, the fare at Temple Street was hearty and included fried bread, sausages and rashers – all no doubt intended to help the girls to stay on their feet.[182] Nevertheless, rigid discipline was enforced and if a nurse arrived late to breakfast four times a month, her day's leave for that month was forfeited. Bríd Joly, who started work as a student nurse in 1969, recalls:

There were five dining areas – the consultant's, the house doctors', the staff nurses and Mrs Foxe's (as it was then known). We took our meals in the student nurses' dining area. It was a very long room and as we came in, we each had to acknowledge the matron. If we were already eating and she came in, we all had to stand up to greet her. As we ate, we had to keep our voices down. You never told the dinner lady that you didn't like a particular food, because she was always sure to pile your plate with it. As we walked out with a 'Good day matron', someone would always be called back. 'Nurse, is there something wrong with your food? You haven't touched it'. She would make you sit down and eat every bit. 'A young girl like you needs to keep her strength up'.[183]

When the girls from the country had finished, they eagerly flocked around the window ledge to see whether there was a letter from home.

By 1893, the sisters were so happy with the quality of their nursing candidates that they decided to buy and fit out No. 13 Temple Street as a home for them. That made it easier for country girls, who no longer had to find accommodation in lodging houses and each room was to be kept in the same manner as if it were in a private residence. In his AGM address of the same year, the Registrar General, Dr Grimshaw, praised the hospital's nurse training programme. He admitted that he had often 'found nurses in his time to attend to sick adults well', but added that 'it was very hard to find nurses who were able to manage sick children properly'.[184]

The following year, the Dublin Metropolitan Technical School for Nurses was established. Each candidate paid one guinea and received a diploma when they passed the examination. By 1898, some Temple Street nurses were even being sent into private practice in an effort to boost hospital revenue. They attended the bedside of sick children in wealthier homes – a service which, according to the mother superior, was available at 'moderate cost'.[185]

When St. Mary's Convalescent Home opened at Cappagh in 1908, young ladies were invited to apply to the superioress at Temple Street to train there as nursery nurses. Instruction was practical and covered the daily care and feeding of children, cookery, laundry, needlework (including cutting out and making clothes), religious teaching for young patients and nursery hygiene. The duration of the course was nine months and the inclusive fee for board, residence and tuition was £20.

In 1919, the State Registration Act was passed. It meant that student nurses were now required to train according to a syllabus laid down by the General Nursing Council (later An Bord Altranais). That included the preliminary state and final sick children's state examinations. Cookery now took second place to classes in anatomy, physiology, hygiene and bacteriology with special courses provided in medical and surgical nursing. Nevertheless, nurses still had to do many labour-intensive jobs such as cleaning down cots and floors and swabbing the operating theatre.

By the 1940s, the career pathway had become increasingly well defined. Every year, about thirty probationers enrolled at

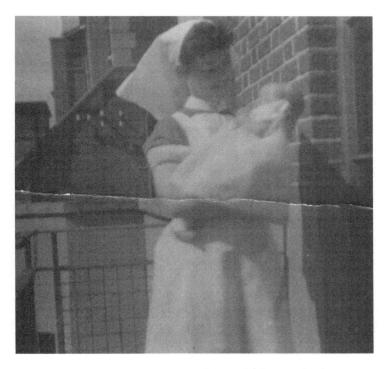

Nurse Josie Curley on the balcony of St. Michael's B ward, July 1959.
(Picture courtesy of Colette Delaney)

Temple Street for preliminary training and of that number, about twenty passed their final exams. Living circumstances were still grim, however, particularly during the winter months when the only form of heating came from a single hearth. Nurse Thomasina Mackey, then twenty years old, recalls:

> This of course was not glowing invitingly as you came off duty tired and cold – the damp turf was there and you spent your two hours' leisure time in an often vain endeavour to light it, or else you retired, defeated, to

your bed – not with a hot water bottle – you were not allowed to boil a kettle in the nurses' home in those days.[186]

Each student had to line up for the doctors in the morning and have all the laboratory results to hand. They were expected to know all the patient records and to carry charts with them. Duty was from 8am to 8pm and they had to be indoors by 9.30pm each night. Smoking in the rooms was forbidden. Occasionally, some sought to break the monotony by attending a dance but, although leave was occasionally given, abuse of the privilege was frowned upon, especially when latecomers were caught sneaking through the ground floor windows. Of one particularly high-spirited probationer, the lady superintendent wrote:

Flighty and uninterested in work. Main reason for nursing appeared to me, to be in City and have a good time. Stayed out late without permission, left hospital door open at 12am while she went on a quest for chip potato[es]. These she had for supper in the ward kitchenette.[187]

On the other hand, there were many things to look forward to. On payday, the nurses all lined up outside the mother superior's office for their brown envelope and there was music and festivities at Christmas with country outings or religious retreats in the summer months. In between times, the nurses found their own way to have fun. Teresa Collins, who worked in St. Michael's block (then across the garden), explains:

I don't know who got the key but we used to let the young Gardaí in from the back lane. We'd give them coffee and sometimes they'd throw their caps up and we'd keep them. Other times, we'd run out to the balcony over the lane and throw the caps back down to them. We were always able to cover our tracks because the block had to be locked separately at night and the night sister used to have to ring over and say that she was coming on her rounds.[188]

In 1954, a new nurses' home called St. Joan's was built on the site of three old houses between the main block and St. George's Church. For the first time, student nurses had access to built-in wardrobes and hot and cold running water and by the early 1970s they no longer had to attend Mass. Nevertheless, discipline was maintained, as Bríd Joly recalls:

The block to the right of the switchboard was for the third year nurses who got a single bedroom to themselves. We weren't so lucky. The home sister was in charge of the young students and there was one telephone on the block – right outside her door which was always kept open. In those days, we received three months of practical training on a mock ward before we were let loose in the hospital but as young nurses we weren't allowed to use the main staircase – we had to use the back stairs and there was a particular order – up on the left; down on the right.

As the century wound to a close, a tunic and trousers replaced the dress and cap of the past. By then, the role of the nurse had evolved considerably. Men were now able to choose nursing as a career and in 2006 a significant link was forged with University College Dublin and Dublin City University with the introduction of the BSc (Nursing) Integrated Children's/General programme. Medical advances had improved survival rates for neonates and children and a new treatment was now available for a range of metabolic disorders. The era of the specialist nurse was born.

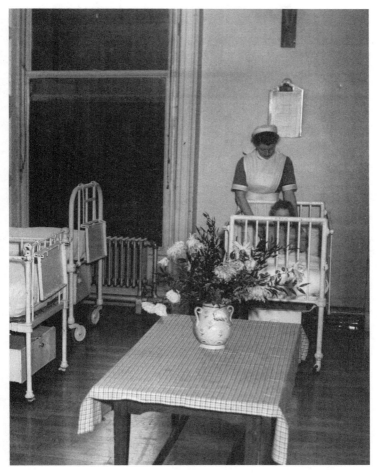

Nurse on her ward round, c.1950. Note the dietary hung over the child's cot.
(Hospital collection)

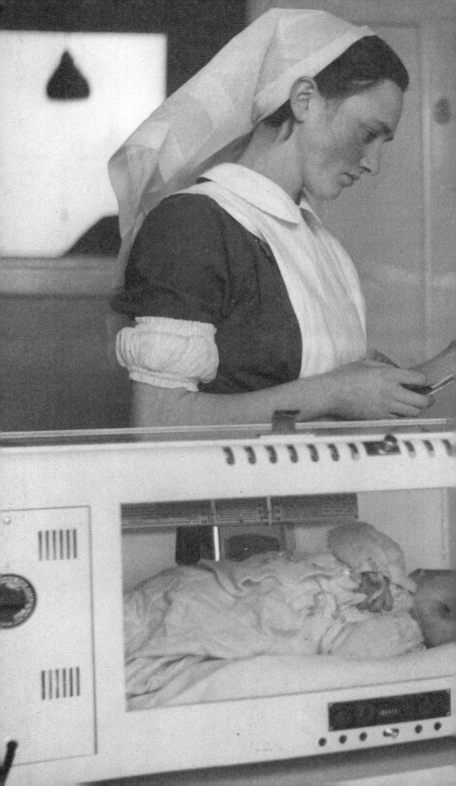

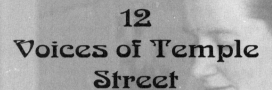

12
Voices of Temple Street

Baby Phyllis Gaffney, pictured here in April/May 1952. She was Temple Street's first incubator baby. In October 1951, her eldest brother died in a drowning accident. Less than three months later, her father was killed in an Aer Lingus plane crash in Snowdonia. As a consequence of her mother's shock, Baby Phyllis stopped gaining weight in utero. When she was born on 30 March 1952 in a nursing home in Galway weighing just 2.5lbs, her grandfather drove her to Temple Street, accompanied by a nurse. She remained an inpatient for four to six weeks.
(Hospital collection)

emple Street Hospital relies on a diverse group of professionals to look after the children in its care. Every day, the service is sustained not just through the efforts of medical personnel but also by the work of canteen staff, hospital porters, household staff, maintenance personnel and administrators, each of whom have their own part to play. In many ways, the hospital is like a small town – home to 1,100 people. These interviews reflect the diversity of the patient and staff experience.

The Emergency Consultant

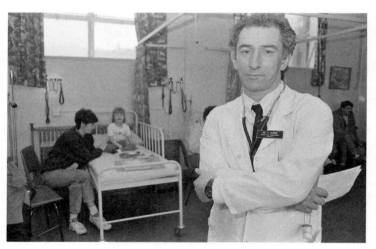

Dr Peter Keenan, 21 March 1991. (Picture courtesy of National Library Photographic Archive)

Dr Peter Keenan (aged sixty-three) is one of Ireland's best-known emergency consultants. Having trained in various hospitals in the UK and Ireland, he was the first doctor to hold a paediatric A&E post in Ireland. He spent twenty-seven years at Temple Street from

1984 to 2011. During that time, he treated everything from bumps and breaks to coughs and colds and witnessed the emergence of a multi-cultural community in the north inner city.

My father was born in a flat on Mountjoy Square in 1913. Afterwards he was reared with his three brothers in Nottingham Street on the North Strand. When he was about eight years old, he and one of his brothers were walked up to Temple Street by their mother via Nerney's Court and into the outpatients department to have their tonsils and adenoids removed under chloroform or ether. His memory of it was that some kind of material – a bandage or cotton wool for soakage – was shoved into his mouth because he was pouring blood. Afterwards, they were put into a horse and trap for the trip back to Nottingham Street.

I was born in 1951. I was also admitted to Temple Street for about a week when I was about four months old. In later years, I found a very brief note in the records that read, 'Five-month-old child – screaming a lot' (familiar symptomatology). The next note read 'circumcision; home'. In other words, if all else fails, do something.

I went to secondary school at Colaiste Mhuire in nearby Parnell Square. While I was there I joined the Legion of Mary and one of the things we did was to bring kids from the local tenements to Mass on Sunday morning in the Pro Cathedral. We also did Sunday morning visitations in Temple Street as part of our 'charitable works'. In those days, parents were told, 'Ok, leave him with us now and don't come to visit'. I can clearly remember being up in St. Patrick's Ward playing with the little toddlers in their iron barred cots.

In 1984, I had started in general practice at Lucan, County Dublin when the first paediatric emergency job in the country was advertised at Temple Street. I knew the hospital well. In 1977, I had worked there as a casualty officer for six months, returning the following year to do another stint as registrar under Professor Niall O'Doherty – a troubled genius and a very entertaining man with a deep interest in inherited syndromes.

When I started in the new consultancy post, they couldn't have fashioned a better job because if I had any kind of gift, it was that I was versatile. Some people are lucky and end up as a round peg in a round hole; in other words, they get a job that really suits them, but a substantial number of the human race are not so fortunate. If I had ended up being a specialist, I might not have been so good at it but I am a bit of a DIY man. I was suited to A&E, where I had to stand back and say, well if I go completely linear with this, it just won't work.

In the beginning, the department was tiny and always packed with people. It was little more than a tiled corridor with people sitting on chairs and a dressing room that had a number of little alcoves in it. You could barely turn – if you needed to go in and stitch something, you had to walk in and reverse out. We were seeing patients two at a time, all the time. At times, you would be sitting at a table talking to a mother and examining a child's chest or ears or throat and a yard behind you, the surgical registrar would be holding down a child who was roaring and screaming as he tried to stitch him up.

In the mornings, I used to park my Ford Anglia beside St. George's Church, but as a precaution I always took the coil out of it. I often came back in the evening time to find a gang of local kids sitting in it. Over the years, I got to know many of them as regular A&E attendees. You'd often have some form of banter with them or their parents based on what kind of relationship you had. When they saw me, some of them would protest, 'Now don't be giving out to me. You threw me out the last time' and I'd say 'I'll throw you out again if you're not careful – very fast'. So we had this adversarial relationship that would be intimate and verbal with a lot of badinage going on.

I was always amazed by Dublin malapropisms. There's a skin infection called impetigo which is caused by bacteria in the skin. In the old days, it used to be called 'school sores'. Time and time again, I explained to the parents:

'He has impetigo.'

The mother would hit her husband on the arm:

'I told you. It's infantago!'

'No', I repeated, 'it's impetigo'.

'I know doctor; he has infantago'.

I grew to love 'infantago' so much I would actually manipulate people to say it.

Then there was the whole mythology of illness. After a seizure, you might hear a mother say, 'I thought he was going to swalley his tongue'. I used to explain that nobody ever swallowed their tongue. It was all rubbish but nevertheless it was a privilege to get the chance to disabuse parents of such misconceptions. Another time, a child would arrive in with a big lump on his head; mother and grandmother in tow. After taking a careful look, I would explain it was unlikely he had a fracture and that there was nothing to suggest he had injured his brain. The grandmother would turn to her daughter and say:

'I told yeh. Once the bump came out the outside; that took the pressure off'.

The reasoning was incredible. It was almost Einsteinian – the dissipation of energy got carried out with the bump. It was all garbage but it made a certain amount of folk sense.

During the late eighties and early nineties, there was a meningitis scare. We saw huge numbers of patients and at one point I was on my feet for a whole weekend. There was a lot of confusion among the general public – the idea that if you had been in contact with somebody who knew somebody else with meningitis, you might catch it.

Then, two children from different halting sites on the fringes of the north city caught it and the travelling community arrived in droves. The laneway down to casualty was chockablock with vans because they had been told by the public health people to come in and get preventative antibiotics. It was completely unnecessary but the travellers were very difficult to reassure – they wanted to have their children seen and it was difficult to send them home so we had to open the assembly hall to accommodate them.

It was a bit like one of those Western movies with Elmer Gantry or Burt Lancaster where people sell snake-oil medicine from covered wagons. I was up on stage trying to address the masses that filled the hall:

'It is really only necessary to have the antibiotic if you had kissing contact'.

It was like a biblical scene with big traveller mothers, fathers and children all over the place. One woman stood with her arms outstretched imploring:

'Doctor, save the children!'

And I shouted back, 'We've run out of antibiotics. We'll have more later on!'

During the 1990s, there was a wave of immigration. Suddenly it wasn't Sean O'Casey's Dublin anymore. By talking to the West Africans I found that some were from ex-French colonies such as the Congo, Cote D'Ivoire, Senegal and I have a bit of French so I enjoyed speaking to them. The other thing I noted was their evangelical Christianity. On one occasion, a Nigerian woman came in with a chesty child. I quickly realised that he had mild asthma, which is a common enough problem. Oftentimes, it is easier for doctors to treat it with antibiotics than to explain that it is a wheezing illness that will come and go. 'What your child has is not an infection', I explained. 'He has been on antibiotics and they are not working. The noise you are hearing in his chest is an obstruction as he tries to get rid of air out of his lungs. This is called asthma'. I got distracted then but when I came back she seemed quite distressed and was chanting something.

'What are you doing?' I asked. 'Are you praying?'

'Yes', she said. 'I am praying doctor. I am saying, Jesus I reject asthma; Jesus, I reject asthma!'

Oftentimes, antibiotics are ineffective but it is uncomfortable to see child who is distressed, particularly at night when everybody loses sleep. It's very hard to tell people: 'it might get worse; it might come back but there's nothing I can give you'. You'd be talking to one family like that and out of the corner of your eye, you could see that the child in the next bed had the same thing. 'Did you hear that?' I used to say. 'Did you hear what I said to that mother? And she'd say, 'Yeah, I was listening ', and I'd say 'Well it's exactly what I'm going to say to you'. That's a very hard message to sell. On the other hand, the tendency to overprescribe has been the driving force of the greatest amount of mythology and garbage as well as putting doctors on pedestals.

When drugs came in, the aftermath was very hard to deal with. It is extraordinary to think that a child might be born to a heroin or methadone-addicted mother and need to be detoxed in the newborn baby unit in the Rotunda using Valium and other drugs and still be shaking from withdrawal symptoms for three weeks until they are feeding OK and not jittery anymore. Then they're handed straight back into the same environment – cold, threadbare, filthy, vermin-infested, nothing but bits of bread and biscuits, no nourishment in the place; the parents bombed out; they really haven't a prayer.

During the early nineties, I attended a conference with one of our social workers in Strasbourg. The Danes were actually talking about taking children away from addicts at birth. Some of the so-called more advanced societies would tell parents: 'We don't think that you are actually fit to be in charge of one of our citizens'.

Today, there is a sense that the child is the possession of the parents and that the state is big brother. I don't think we serve the newborn citizen very well in terms of what we allow and the problem is that smaller children have no voice. That sounds very sentimental but it is true. The hardwiring that goes on in the brain during the first year of life is crucial – making eye contact, smiling back at you, being able to recognise a stranger from people you know, responding to love and touch and affection, frowns versus smiles – these are not just behavioural things that every child does; these are actually laid down by neurons migrating in your brain under stimulus and if that doesn't happen by the age of one, it's all over. If your parents were bombed out and hadn't been playing coochie coo, cuddling you and making eye contact, the opportunity to connect one part of the brain to the other is lost.

We expect children to grow up as functioning members of society with a sense of civic responsibility; with the ability to love and a willingness to share and interact with others – it's a tough gig for the best advantaged children.

Recently, I was walking near where I live in Phibsborough when a woman and her husband recognised me:

'Why aren't you down there working?' they said.

'Ah', I said, 'I've given up'.

'We went down to you for years. They're all grown up now'.

I still get a lot of that.

Life is an incurable disease that ends in death for every single one of us and the verbal vehicle that joins that journey from cradle to grave is made up of science, mythology, opportunism of all sorts; the comic and the tragic. You come across it all in A&E.

The Nurse

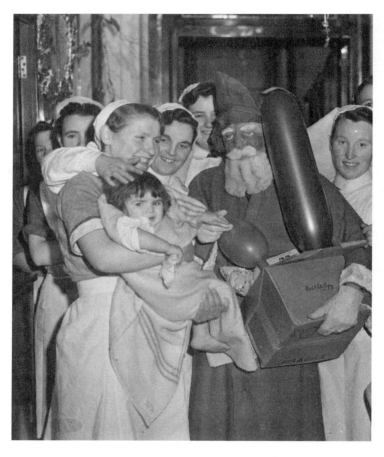

Nurse Annie Funge (holding Lawrence Kenny) with Santa, 28 December 1950. (Hospital collection)

Annie Bernadette Funge (aged eighty-two) comes from Gorey, County Wexford. She joined Temple Street as a young probationer in June 1949. Here, this 'refined, gentle nurse' (as her file records) recalls the atmosphere at the hospital during the post-war years when poverty was rife, none of the instruments were disposable and students were expected to learn on the job. Arriving from the country, she was told of the night of the terrible bombing of the North Strand which shook the hospital windows.

I was born in Gorey, County Wexford in 1932 where my father worked as an insurance agent. I went to school at the Loreto Convent and when I turned sixteen, I decided that I would like to train as a nurse in Temple Street. Before being accepted, I had to attend an interview with the matron. That consisted of a written and oral test as well as a medical examination under Dr Kavanagh. When I was accepted as a probationer, I was told to go to the Sisters of Charity convent in Stanhope Street for my uniform – it consisted of a dress with removable white sleeves, an apron, a cap and black-laced shoes with heavy, grey lisle stockings. The removable sleeves had to be worn everywhere outside the ward and for doing the doctors' rounds. We were not allowed to wear make-up or jewellery – not even the tiniest earring – and we had to carry a pocket watch with a second hand so that we could check pulse and respiration rates.

All nurses, staff and students alike, lived in and we had no choice in the matter. At first, we were given four-bedded rooms, eventually sharing two-bedded accommodation but there was no en suite and we were not allowed to smoke. Once, when a student who smoked gave her word of honour that she did not, she was expelled; not for smoking but for giving her word of honour. Matron told us afterwards that if we did not have our word of honour, we had nothing. Uniform was so important and punctuality went without saying. No talking or running on corridors: 'Run only on case of fire or haemorrhage'. We were never allowed to address anyone by their Christian name and most definitely not the doctors.

There were three sitting rooms, each with a coal fire burning daily from autumn to the end of spring. The fires were attended to by the cleaning staff and a supply of coal left in each sitting room.

On the first day, we just put on our uniforms and went straight to work. There was no prior training – you just learnt as you went along and woe betide you if you were not smart and observant. The matron, Miss Sharkey, was responsible for our education and behaviour and she demanded the highest standards and absolute correctness. She was a superb disciplinarian but she also strived to impart good qualities.

Every morning, we were called at six o'clock and we had to be in the chapel at half past for prayers. If the bell rang before we arrived, we were marked late. Two late marks in a month meant that we had to work on one of our days off until nine in the morning (we had just two days off every month with two half days). We had our breakfast at seven and went on duty at half seven. If we were on night duty, we had no choice but to attend lectures the following morning before going to bed.

The work was hard and we never had money to spare, yet we had no shopping, housework or bills to worry about. A cause of some amusement was when Matron would say, 'Girls, you came here to do nursing; not O'Connell Street'.

Every day, we had our own routine – beds and lockers were pulled out from the wall so that the ward maid could clean every inch of the floor. We wiped everything with carbolic solution, including beds, tables, lockers and surfaces. Stainless steel and glass trollies were cleaned with methylated spirit and when that was done, there was the bathroom, toilet and sluice room to attend to. When a child was taken to theatre, we had to strip the entire bed, clean the area again with carbolic solution and make it up with clean linen.

Absolutely nothing was disposable but central sterilisation of equipment was unheard of. Instead, we had an electric steriliser on each ward. We boiled all our instruments, syringes and needles but that meant that a lot of work prior to setting up IV drips, lumbar punctures and daily injections. There was a certain amount of anxiety involved. We had to keep checking the needles because constant boiling and banging around in the steriliser made them blunt. When the equipment was ready, we used a long cheatle forceps to take them out of the boiling water.

We were surrounded by tenements, said to be the worst in Europe. After coming off night duty, it was quite common to be woken the following afternoon by sounds from the street. The rag and bone man with his horse and cart came by frequently calling, 'Rags, bottles, jam jars – come down when you're ready', and the women in the tenements brought down odds and ends for which they were paid a small sum of money. Another familiar sound came from children in the street. They played skipping games to rhymes such as:

Nursie, nursie I am sick,

Send for the doctor quick, quick, quick,

Doctor, doctor shall I die?

Yes my child, so shall I.

Another one went:

I see a little nurse,

And she is not too tall,

You see her every day sitting in the hall,

Her uniform is blue and her veil is white,

She is my darling day and night.

Patients were admitted from all over the country. Our Lady's Hospital, Crumlin had not yet opened and Temple Street was the main hospital for children. Times were very poor, however, and many did not have their own transport. There was never any facility for family members to stay and many children arrived by ambulance on their own; visiting hours had to be strictly adhered to and we never had the assistance of a relative to give emotional support to those who were away from home.

Because of the poverty and dreadful living conditions in the tenements, there was a constant flow of very ill babies suffering from gastroenteritis, upper respiratory infection and pneumonia. A very important part of our duty was to inspect each head for lice twice a day. I don't remember any special treatment other than swabbing with Dettol solution and fine combing over and over again. The most distressing illness we had to deal with was tuberculosis – most especially TB meningitis because the treatment was so very harsh. When the children saw a nurse coming, they used to scream because they had to administer streptomycin deep into the muscles every four hours and the prognosis was very poor. Night duty was very tough in the baby unit with not a minute to spare all night long. After finishing my shift, I often fell asleep in the bath and only woke up when the water got cold.

I went on to do all my general training with the Sisters of Mercy in St. John's and St. Elizabeth in London. There, I was told by one of the nuns that they really liked getting Temple Street nurses because of the great training we had received. I still remember one sunny morning as I crossed the garden on my way to St. Michael's unit – the bells rang out from nearby St. George's Church. It was a heavenly moment.

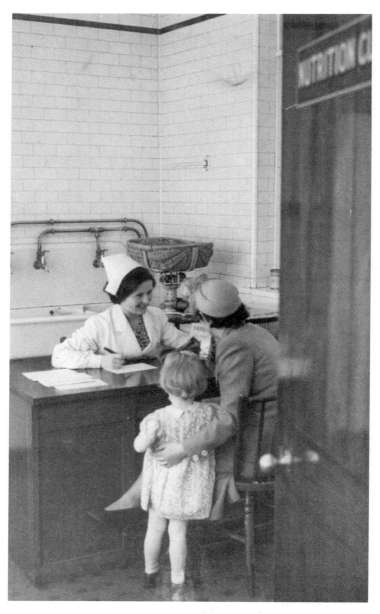

Kitty Randles, who became Temple Street's first dietician in 1950.
(Hospital archive)

The Dietician

Catherine (Kitt) Randles (aged eighty-five) from County Kerry was Temple Street's first dietician. She arrived there as a young, spirited girl in 1950, keen to make her mark. It was an optimistic time. As she herself remarks, she saw herself as an educated lady working towards 'a new Ireland'. On the other hand, she was challenged on two fronts – the poverty that surrounded the hospital and entrenched attitudes to dietary management among hospital staff. Then, as now, the patient was central to everything.

I was born in Kenmare, County Kerry and went to school as a border in St. Louis, Monaghan. During the war years, we were given a small suitcase packed with our pyjamas, toothpaste and other essentials in case Monaghan got a stray bomb. I came to Dublin around 1944 to train as a dietician in Cathal Brugha Street and lived with a few others in Mountjoy Square. Afterwards I went to work in Great Ormond Street, London.

Rose Simmons, who was the lady in charge there, asked me to take a letter over to Dublin to a dietetics sister in St. Vincent's Hospital, St. Stephen's Green. Dietetics had only started in Ireland and there were very few jobs available. Unknown to me, Ms Simmons had described me glowingly in the letter as 'Grand Ms Randles' and on foot of that, I was invited to an interview with the reverend mother in Vincent's. She asked me would I go down to Temple Street. I thought it was a bit out of my way but I went anyway.

At that time, Dr Dundon was on the Temple Street staff. He had been in America where he saw that dietetics was a growing profession. Patients were being sent home from Temple Street with nothing more than a diet sheet from their doctor and no follow up; the medical board was concerned and Dr Dundon said he wouldn't return to work unless a service was started on the same lines. For me, it was a case of being in the right place at the right time.

I met the reverend mother and the bursar in September 1950. They asked me if I was confident enough to start up a new department so I said that I would and I got the job. At that time the hospital was more like an old house – very upstairs/downstairs and we had a very pretty garden where the nuns used to sit during their two-hour break. My department was in the basement; I just about managed to get a corner beyond the old milk kitchen that had been set up some years before by an Austrian lady – a sister-in-law to one of the doctors.

In the beginning, they didn't know what to do with me but I was given a very nice room to sleep in up behind St. Philomena's Ward. I ate with the housemen, Lily Butler, our hospital manager and the pharmacist, who was a widow. The nurses ate in the dining room where they were watched over strictly by the matron. One of them told me, 'You'll have to get permission to be out later than ten o'clock'. When they were coming back in after an evening out, they used to advise each other as a kind of cant to put a bit of lipstick on before they met the matron. She knew you were courting if you had no lipstick on.

On one occasion, I went to ask Mr Mowbray about staying out at night – I knew I could twist him around my little finger:

'Who do I have to get permission from to go out to the pictures?'

'What do you mean?'

'Well the nurses have to get permission'.

'You don't need it', he said. 'If anyone asks, just tell them I gave it to you'.

After that, I used to go out frequently. The home warden used to ask, 'Ms Randles, are you in or out tonight?' I used to say I was staying in, even if I wasn't because that meant that a fire would always be lighting in my bedroom. When I came back late I used to give a cheery smile to the night sister, which I would say she resented!

Having arrived from Great Ormond Street, I was shocked to find that mothers were feeding their babies on bottles of warm tea. They didn't have the milk and there was awful starvation. At the same time, the father would get his Guinness and the mother her cigarettes. I used to spend my Saturday mornings with the Jesuits and the Legion of Mary doing penny dinners for local people in Summerhill. During the week, we used to go and beg bits of meat from the butchers in the market and fill jam jars and paint pots with stew for them.

I shared a divided room in the outpatient department with our almoner, Sr Francis Regis. We saw patients from all over the country but a lot came from Dublin. Together, we implemented a food scheme to help the poorest families. We struck a deal with a shop in Dorset Street and when I wrote out the diet for the parents to follow, Sr Regis would give them a voucher. That helped to ensure that they couldn't use it on cigarettes or beer.

TB was a big thing and we saw a lot of children with rickets which was associated with it. I was keen to introduce dietary management of disease. During the war, the Dutch had discovered that gluten in bread affected those with coeliac disease but I had to be very diplomatic with some of the older doctors when I told them that they shouldn't be giving their patients toast. One day, one of the surgeons, Mr Shanley, asked me, 'Tell me now, do you believe in this Vitamin C in orange juice before surgery?' 'Oh yes', I said. 'That's used in a lot of hospitals in England'. Taking my advice, Mr Shanley decided to follow suit because there was a belief that it would help to heal wounds quicker. It had to be freshly squeezed rather than in pill form. When I asked the nun in charge of the pantry for twelve oranges, she was shocked. She just said, 'Oh, they're very expensive'.

When I got married in December 1954, I had to leave work as that was the custom for women in those days. St. Vincent's had started up an internship for dieticians but it had only been in operation for four months when the poor old nun in charge got sick. I was sent for in January and asked whether I would train the students. They had four years of college at Cathal Brugha Street and six months' practice. I explained that I was a married woman and that my husband was used to his lunch in the middle of the day. 'Oh that's all right dear', they said. 'You can arrange your lectures around that'. I accepted the post but I used to go back to my home in Mespil Flats during the afternoon, make my husband lunch, do the washing up and go back to take the students up to the Coombe for their maternity training.

I spent just four years at Temple Street but it will always remain in my heart. The hospital was like a miniature town with a wonderful spirit of cooperation. I can't emphasise that enough. The nuns were workaholics but I was too; we got on well together.

They did it for God whereas I was doing it for a New Ireland. I saw myself as a privileged young girl who had been trained in a profession. Then, as now, the patient was what mattered. That's the way it should be.

The Porter

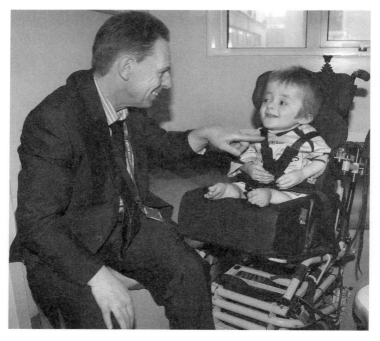

Head Porter John Doyle pictured with Michael Stokes, November 2011.
(Picture taken by Brian McEvoy for TV3)

During an average year, each Temple Street porter walks an astonishing 1,000 miles up corridors and stairs in their effort to deliver essential services. Head porter John Doyle is no exception. During his thirty-four years at the hospital, he has literally travelled in the footsteps of his father who did the same job before him for over fifty years. 'Temple Street,' he says, 'is like a good jacket that fits well on the shoulder blades.'

I was born in Marlborough Street in the heart of Dublin city where the Eircom building stands now. When I was just three years old, we moved to Cabra which was a sprawling new suburb. One of my earliest memories of Temple Street was a two-day stay in St. Patrick's Ward where the food was boiled mince that didn't taste very nice.

My dad had been an inner city man all his life and he came to work here as a porter in 1941 during the Second World War. At that time, the hospital was very much an upstairs/downstairs kind of building where you understood your place and you didn't get in people's way.

One of the jobs my dad and Tom Cobbe had to do was to clean out the fires on a regular basis. At that time, the old coal bunkers were still filled at the front of the hospital and for them, it was like having to be a stoker on a ship or a train – they had to keep the place going through summer and winter. There were five or six parlours, including the nuns' community room, and they all had fireplaces. As soon as they were all set, the men would go off, have a wash and present themselves for breakfast at nine o'clock, but they had to demonstrate to the nuns that they had clean hands and a clean face before they were fed. There was no such thing as them turning up saying, 'Look at me, I'm Al Jolson'.

Probably the most distinctive thing about Temple Street back then was the antiseptic smell. It denoted cleanliness and you would even see nurses down on their knees cleaning floors on a regular basis.

I also remember my dad telling me about himself and Tom Cobbe on the hospital roof, hanging flags of celebration out. Significantly, everybody in the hospital fifty years ago was on call at all times and it was unheard of to say, 'I'm going home at four o'clock and can't be contacted'. There was a real family atmosphere and everybody played a part.

Temple Street Children's Hospital

I started working here slightly after my twenty-first birthday. Back then, I had no intention of making it my career. I had been working in the bar trade so I thought I might take a break and weigh up my options. I had a ten-minute interview with the hospital manager Ms Lily Butler, who asked me what I had been doing and where I was working. She finished by wishing me well and hoped I would enjoy my time in Temple Street.

Coming to work here, you very quickly learned that it was a system that worked on routine and everyone understood their role. We used to have to do the brasses on the front door and clean the fireplaces on a regular basis. There was also a wooden board in the front hall that had little metal plates with the names of all on-call consultants on it. The list had to be right or questions would be asked. We also kept a paper record of all the inpatients who were in the hospital. Between times, we carried linen baskets of laundry up the stairs and when a light bulb blew on a ward, we had to change it – it's amazing how many of the lads had to get someone to hold the ladder for them because they thought the bulb was going to blow and they'd end up going through the roof.

Every job has a quirky side and in Temple Street, it was the custom for the consultants to get their cup of tea (coffee was a rarity) at 11am every morning with a plate of fresh biscuits. The boardroom was hallowed ground and you never called a doctor by their first name.

One morning, I was sitting at the front desk having a smoke when I sensed a presence standing beside me. No words were exchanged. Next, I heard the sound of hands rubbing together. As a naive young man, I didn't know what the gesture meant but in the boldness of youth, I turned to find Professor Kavanagh standing there:

'Can I help you Professor?'

'Young Doyle, is today a black fast day?'

'No, I don't think so Professor.'

'Well that's very good', he said, 'because I'd like to know when I'm going to get my cup of tea this morning'.

By the time I started at Temple Street, the boilers were running on oil and it was our job to make sure they were kept filled. Otherwise they would sit down. That entailed pumping probably 500 gallons of oil into them but it took us a long time to understand the rhythm of left, right – like a rocking chair. When the older porters took over, they made it look very easy but being young and naive, if the job took forty minutes, we would want to do it in fifteen to get it over with. We'd go hell for leather but after a couple of minutes, the heat would start to take its toll and the job would end up taking two hours. It was the 1980s version of a Jacuzzi – you went in with your jacket on and came out as if you were after doing a workout.

Thirty-four years on, I fully appreciate the role my late father had in the hospital; at the start of my journey I thought that all I had to do was walk behind him and that I didn't have to do a lot. I soon realised that before I could walk in his footsteps, I had to demonstrate the same values that he had.

In more recent years, support services have developed to the point where we now interact more with other health workers. All of us are involved in patient care. You tend to become more engaged with some children due to the complex nature of their illnesses, but no matter how professional you try to be, there are always some who pull at the heartstrings. Some never made it out of Temple Street but twenty years on, you still remember them.

Temple Street Children's Hospital

Some of the changes I have seen are for the better. Visiting wasn't a common practice even thirty years ago, but today we encourage parents take their place at the bedside. The bond between families can never be broken; we are here to provide care but at times we become a second family to the patient.

Today, when I look at everything that goes on around me, I still marvel at the professionalism shown to our patients. You have to sit at a bedside to see it in action. It comes from the heart. I feel very glad to be part of that team. Like a good jacket, it fits comfortably around the shoulder blades.

Temple Street is a hospital but it is also home to a unique family who even today call it the 'house'. Family, past and present, has always been at the centre of what makes that house a home; it is one of the main reasons why we love and believe in what we do.

The Lab Scientist

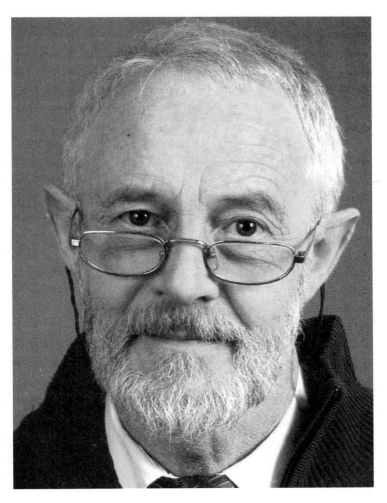

Ray O Ceallaigh. (Picture courtesy of Tommy Nolan)

Ray O Ceallaigh (aged seventy-one) started work at Temple Street as a junior laboratory assistant in 1964. Here, he recalls his early experiences working in a department which in some ways was quite basic but in others embodied the hospital's pioneering spirit of scientific advancement.

I was born and raised in Clontuskert, just a few miles outside Ballina. My parents were farmers and I was the eldest of nine so further education was not an option. When I finished secondary school in Ballinasloe, I had to start looking for a job. Some of the girls in our area might have got work in the civil service but most of the boys ended up in America or England. I spent the summer before my Leaving Cert in London – it seemed like the whole parish was there. Afterwards, I came to Dublin where I got a couple of clerical jobs but I didn't like them. I just wanted to do something with my hands.

I was working for a company called Milner's in Lombard Street, doing sums about how much so many lengths of steel would cost when I spotted a small newspaper ad for a job in the laboratory in Temple Street. There was no application form. I just wrote a letter saying I was interested and that was it. One Saturday morning, I was interviewed in the parlour by Ms Butler and by the head of the laboratory, Dr Seamus Cahalane. Everything was quite informal. 'Can you start on Monday?' 'Yes.' 'Great'. There was no paperwork – just my name and address. This was just one year after doing the Leaving Cert.

When I started, there were only seven of us. The department was quite open plan, comprising microbiology, biochemistry as well as histology, which was run from one little corner by Mr Joly. A kind of long office housed haematology, blood transfusion and Dr Cahalane's room. He was a young and ambitious scientist who had come back from America. We also had a good woman called Mrs Flanagan who used to wash and sterilise the urine bottles, clean them and attach all the labels. The nurses used to bring those bottles back to us with the samples in them.

The work was manual and very smelly at times. We used the kind of equipment you would see in old books – retort tubes, bottles and gas Bunsens with tripods over them. It was a primitive type of science. Looking back on it now, it was almost like a school laboratory. You read the textbook and did the tests listed in it. That book could be sixty years old but the tests were still considered valid. We used to make our own pipettes by melting a glass tube over the Bunsen and drawing it out to the right length. We also lit our cigarettes and pipes over the gas flame. New equipment was very expensive and it would have gone into other hospitals before it came to us.

A lady called Nancy who worked in St. Michael's C Ward used to bring us tea and biscuits every day on a tray with a pot covered by a cosy. She used to wheel it down into the middle of the microbiology department where we had a table. Sometimes samples would be left alongside it.

Throughout the day, we visited the wards to perform full blood counts. That involved making a skin prick, sucking the blood into a tube and stoppering it. If you were in the ward at noon or six in the evening, you had to stand and say the Angelus before carrying on with your work. The nuns had their sleeping quarters at the top of the house. One evening, as I came down the corridor with Mr Joly, who was smoking his pipe, an elderly sister stopped us and said, 'You know you shouldn't be smoking here; this is a convent'.

There was a piggery at the end of the casualty lane and on a really hot summer, the smell was awful – it would permeate the whole place. You'd hear the pigs squealing when they were being fed. Alongside that was a blacksmith's forge. When the farrier was shoeing horses, you'd get the smell of the molten hoof as he matched the shoe to it.

At that time, live-in staff such as the nuns, doctors and nurses had their own separate dining areas. We had nowhere to eat so we took our lunch in the lab or went out. When it came to the nurses, the matron usually sat near enough to the refectory entrance. As the students came in, they had to bow to her before they took their seats. We used to organise a couple of dances in the old outpatients department for them but the assembly hall was better because it had a wooden floor. I didn't date too many nurses though, because they couldn't be out later than ten o'clock and the porter would be waiting above in the hall where they had to sign in on a book.

Another thing I remember was the old Antonian Missionary Press which was based at the back of the hospital. It had two people working in it – Billy and Joe. They sold everything you might find in a missionary stall – beads, prayer books, leaflets, medals and holy water, not to mention *St. Anthony's Annals* which were sent all over the world from those Dickensian offices – old and musty with poor lighting.

We tested for the common things – colds, flus, tonsillitis; mostly fairly simple illnesses. A few studies had been done elsewhere on asymptomatic urinary tract infections and Dr Cahalane decided that we should follow suit. I had a scooter which I used to go out to the schools and collect the glass bottles. We made a little square box with Styrofoam in it to hold them. Arrangements were made with each school to collect the samples and my job was to take them back to the lab and test them. In those days, the children had a catchphrase: 'No bottles, no milk', but when they saw me arriving, some of them used to shout, 'No bottles, no pee!' Once I was coming down the North Circular Road when all of a sudden a car turning left knocked me off the bike. I wasn't hurt but it must have been priceless to see me running to get the full sample bottles as they rolled all over the road.

We did our TB work in the middle of the lab. There was no partition and no safety cabinets; the air could easily fly around with the bacilli in it. I thought it was crazy but there wasn't an awful lot I could do about it. I know people who worked in laboratories who actually got the disease but thankfully nobody ever caught it in Temple Street. When I expressed my concern, I was told, 'Well even if you get it, won't you be alright? The Health Department will look after you'.

Our agar plates used to go into the incinerator chimney on the hospital grounds. The same chimney was used to burn any papers that might have been left around but oftentimes, half-burned documents would sail right up through the chimney and land in George's Pocket behind the hospital. It was a frequent occurrence for people to call in to notify the hospital that some charred letter or other had been discovered.

I met Bob Guthrie once or twice when he came over from the United States. He seemed to be a nice man; he had arrived to help set up the new screening service for newborn infants. We had decided to test for a metabolic disease called Phenylketonuria – it meant that an enzyme called phenylalanine was missing and it resulted in many people being institutionalised for mental health deficiencies. Mr Joly used to work on the blood spot samples that came in from the maternity hospitals. He'd put the blood spots onto an agar plate and then do a test to show the level of Phenylalanine in the blood. Then they began to discover a few cases so they extended it and in the end there could have been eight, ten or twelve plates before they moved over to the new system. Now the technology is so great, you can even do genetics on blood spots and the range of tests has hugely expanded.

When I started at Temple Street, everybody accepted that they fitted into a certain stratum but at the same time, the hospital was a motherly kind of place where the nuns took care of the junior nurses. Every Christmas we used to get a present from the sister in charge – enough cloth to make a skirt for the girls whereas the lads got a cap, gloves or a scarf. Today, things are different in some ways but there is still a warm family atmosphere – thankfully that hasn't changed much.

The Maintenance Manager

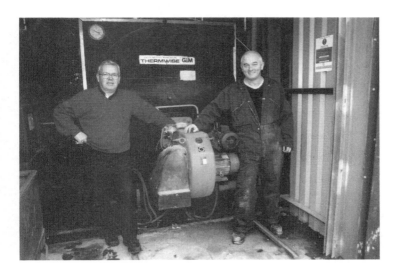

Maintenance Manager Jack Kennerk, pictured with Plumber, Willie
Malone, 2001. (Hospital collection)

*Maintenance is an often unseen aspect of hospital life. Here, retired
departmental manager Jack Kennerk (aged seventy-four) describes
his work at Temple Street in an era before Celtic Tiger prosperity.
With few resources at their disposal, he and his crew ensured that
essential services were kept running behind the scenes.*

I come from a family of seven children. We were raised in
Henrietta Street Flats before moving up to Auburn Street where
my mother ran a grocery shop. She kept Rhode Island Reds out
the back and we used to collect the eggs from them. My father
was a commercial traveller.

As a baby, I was admitted to Temple Street twice in 1940
with broncho-pneumonia. I was taken over from Henrietta

Street and put up in Camillus' Ward and then St. Michael's. Visiting was very restricted in those days – parents and visitors would stand on the pavement outside, waving up at their children.

My next experience of Temple Street started in 1989. I had been working with FÁS as a foreman on renovation projects such as the Tailor's Hall and St. Anne's Church on Dawson Street and I was invited to renovate an old parish building called George's Hall. It later became the consulting rooms for Nephrologist Professor Denis Gill.

Up until that point, Professor Gill had been working in a small Portakabin at the end of the hospital garden with rotten chipboard floors and steps that didn't even have a handrail. Privately, Mother Superior Sr Anne Eucharia described him as a saint to work in those conditions.

At that time, the local area had a lot of problems with drugs. Hospital staff had to be chaperoned by porters when they went to their cars at night and thieves used to come in and steal the public telephones off the walls. To remedy that, I got quarter-inch-thick metal plates made to bolt the phones onto. When an engineer came up to fit one of the replacements he said, 'What's all this metal for? This place is like Fort Knox'. He couldn't believe it when I told him that people were actually stealing the phones. 'But this is a hospital', he kept saying. Things got so bad that the local residents barred off both ends of the Hardwicke Street Flats to get rid of the drug pushers. They stood there day and night for three months burning timber in barrels.

One morning, we were having a meeting upstairs in George's Hall when a thief smashed the architect's car window and took his briefcase and coat. When the architect banged on the window, he just looked up, gave him the two fingers and calmly walked away. Afterwards, someone told him he could have his stuff back but it was going to cost him.

While the renovation work was still going on, the personnel manager asked me whether I knew anyone who might do some work. A nurses' inspection was due and they needed somebody to fix a handle on a door or put up some tiles. I was happy to help out and one thing led to another. I was asked to come to work for the hospital as maintenance supervisor (a new post for the hospital). I started on a six-month temporary contract but was later made permanent.

One of the first people I spoke to was a friend in FÁS but when I told him it was a nine-to-four job, he laughed. 'In your dreams', he said, 'I've a brother doing something similar and he never gets home'.

We all have a PhD in hindsight!

My team consisted of a contractor electrician, a plumber, a plumber's helper and a carpenter called Tommy Shiels. The plumber's helper was also the hospital boiler attendant. He was so fond of oranges he was actually able to wallpaper one of the boiler house walls with Jaffa stickers. One Stephens's Day, the drains were badly blocked in Kelly's Row. The drain man was working down the manhole and you could just about see his head. The boiler man stood over him peeling one of his favourite Jaffas. When I arrived, he offered half of it to me with black, oily hands.

'Ah no', I said, 'I don't want to ruin my appetite for dinner'.

Then he offered it to the bloke in the manhole, who took it in his bare hands.

'And would you like an apple?' he said after a minute.

'Ah lovely', the drain man said. 'I'll have that later', and he stuck it in his pocket.

Our carpenter Tommy looked after a huge area on his own. If he wanted a new box of screws, he would have to go to personnel for approval. Without resources, he used to straighten every nail, collect every screw, hinge and lock, and put them in little glass jars for recycling. If he wanted to put a slip on a unit, he would work on it in his little workshop. He used to tell the nurses, 'I'll be getting around to you; you're on the list'. When I questioned him one day about this famous list, he said, 'I do be just telling them that. There's no such thing; it's all in me head'.

For the first year, we had very little resources and my office was out of the back of my car. We had a small little workshop in a Portakabin at the back in the garden with rotten floors. We stored our plywood and timber there and everything was hand-cut – we didn't even have an electric saw.

There were two hospital boilers. One of them ran on medium oil which had been upgraded from coal and the other was run on town gas. The one on medium oil was so old and antiquated that the oil would set like treacle in the burner when it wasn't running. To get it started, you had to throw in lighted rags to melt the oil which could take about five hours. It was most unreliable and sometimes the hospital would have no heat for several hours. Once a year, each boiler had to be shut down, stripped and rebuilt for an insurance inspection which could take up to one week. That meant that the other unreliable boiler would have to be nursed throughout.

Part of my job was to maintain the convent as well because the heating and hot water was supplied from the hospital boilers. You always knew that Sr Eucharia meant business when she put her hands on her hips, as I once found out. She asked me to put a dado rail in one of the convent parlours because the furniture was damaging the walls and we got talking about my job.

'Most people can only keep three things in their head at any one time', she said.

'Well, I have to keep nine or ten in mine', I said. 'I have to think about architects, contractors, maintenance; you name it'.

She seemed impressed. The next day, she called me back.

'Do you remember how you said you were able to keep ten things in your head?'

'Yes', I replied.

'Well', she said, 'you got the wrong room'.

Lift rescue was also part of our job. We couldn't leave the hospital during lunch breaks in case a person got stuck. One night, an engineer was working on the lift when he got trapped between two floors. I was called in at four o'clock in the morning to get him out.

In the early days, I used to do odd jobs for the sisters. I used to arrange a complete maintenance of their headquarters in Donnybrook and I recommended various contractors. One job I organised was a large cleaning area at the back of the kitchens. I arranged for a man to tile the area with a terracotta tile. He used porous ones and when he grouted them, it went into all the pores and instead of terracotta they turned out white. That put me in the bad books with Sr Eucharia and the hands went on the hips again.

In the latter stages, the nuns used to ask me to go for their Easter Palm and put up their Christmas tree. They used to hide the chocolate when I was coming to do bits of maintenance because they knew I had a sweet tooth. From time to time, you could hear them ask, 'Did anyone tell Jack that today is a holy day?'

We often had to deal with gales and storms. One evening, about six corrugated sheets blew off one of the water tanks on the roof. They were eight foot by two and could have easily taken off like Frisbees into Temple Street. The next day, the hairs stood up on the back of my neck when I saw that they all ended up under the tank.[189] Another night, a ten-foot cast-iron chimney toppled into the casualty lane near the front of the house and exploded like a hand grenade, taking down gutters and everything with it. It was a miracle that nobody walked past.

In the early days, we lost water pressure on a regular basis because Dublin City Council had a lot of leaking pipes. A low level water alarm used to go off at the switchboard at night and we would have to call the fire brigade; they would connect their hoses to hydrants in George's Pocket and the casualty laneway. We used to hoist them up to the roof with ropes and fill the tank, which could take four hours.

The guy who came in with me was entitled to go home and get his full sleep but I had to be in my office by eight o'clock the next morning. Depending on which tradesmen had been called out, sometimes I might be carrying three bleeps the following day. I was in the convent one day when I met Tommy the carpenter going up in the lift:

'I could sleep on broken bottles, I feel so lashed out of it', I said. He just looked at me and said, 'I've been feeling like that for the past ten years'.

During my time at the hospital, the mortuary was quite stark and cold – terrazzo floors, tiled walls, green baize, steel presses and marble slabs. I was asked by the bereavement committee to submit a proposal. My plan was to carpet it, lower the ceiling and break it into three sections – a private, peaceful room for the bereaved, an area to gather and make a cup of tea and a centre room for mourners to gather before the removal. Dimmable lighting and carpets went in; I put in air conditioning and took out all the old marble altars. When we were finished, the contrast couldn't be more apparent. We had achieved what we set out to do.

Another large project I was involved with was our backup generator. The old model had to be started by hand and was only able to keep the theatre lights going for twenty minutes (provided of course that you shed the theatre lifts and the rest of the lights in the hospital). In 2000, we installed a full capacity, diesel-powered generator which covered the entire hospital for the first time with enough fuel to keep us going for five days. The work was completed on a Thursday evening and the following Saturday I received a call to say that the generator had kicked in. 'Here we go', I thought, 'teething problems'. I assumed that there had been a fault with the installation until the ESB informed us that a mains cable had been cut in Dorset Street; it would take about an hour and a half to fix. It made me shiver to realise what could have happened if we hadn't finished putting in the new generator on time.

After that, the hospital continued to grow. With the addition of an MRI and CT scanner and extensions and improvements to wards like ICU, we had to upgrade the backup generator in seven years from 600kvi to 1250kvi. I was a hands-on guy who worked in an era before e-mails. I took my job seriously to the extent that I was there day and night and I had to know my job inside out. Looking back on it now, I think there had to be an angel looking after us.

The Community Worker

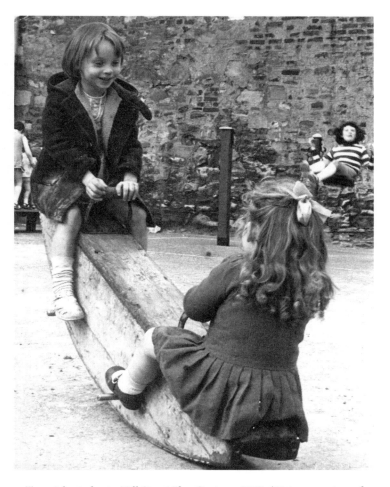

Two girls at play in Hill Street Play Centre, c.1970. (Picture courtesy of
Marie T. Barry)

*Marie T. Barry spent several happy years working at a play centre in
Hill Street. Although she grew up just four miles away from Temple
Street, coming into the inner city was like another world. In her words,
the local community was a 'little hub' of its own. Not only did locals*

take their children to the hospital; many of them also worked there too. Marie got to know many of them over the years. She recalls the difficulties they faced on a day-to-day basis and the fateful events of 17 May 1974, when bombs brought devastation to the city centre.

I started working in Hill Street Play Centre in the early 1970s. My background was social studies and I followed that up with community development; getting involved in play and youth work. I did that as a student which helped to finance my studies; it introduced me to the culture of the people and the problems they had in the inner city. Then I went in and managed the play centre service in Hill Street full time for Dublin City Council.

I grew up in Glasnevin but coming into the North Inner City was like a different world. It was a little hub within a community. The people around Temple Street lived in a small enclave and then you had George's Pocket which was a little entity all on its own.

I started work in the area prior to the Gregory Deal and the tenements in Sean MacDermott Street, Buckingham Street and Summerhill were very much like what you might see in *Strumpet City* – people were still living in sub-divided houses but they did their best.[190] I remember one family who used to collect slops to feed the pigs and they used to run their horses on the beach.

A lot of the kids I worked with would have used Temple Street Hospital quite a lot rather than going to the local GP. He was a great man but the first port of call for all ailments big or small was the hospital. One day I noticed that a boy from Sean MacDermott Street was limping badly; his little foot was sore and he couldn't walk properly so I decided to take him to Temple Street just as the locals did. God knows where his mother and father were. The casualty staff had to strip him down completely.

A doctor came out screaming, 'Where are that child's parents?' He berated me and told me that septicaemia was just about to set in. 'I'm sorry', I said, 'I'm not his mother. I just brought him up for treatment'. The doctor was terribly apologetic. Afterwards I brought the boy home having promised that I would bring him back; the parents were so crazy. It was a very tragic situation.

Yet some of the kids did extremely well. A lot of the local mothers were employed by the hospital in Temple Street. They were wonderful. After a day's work, they used to tell me, 'Yer wan tests afterwards to see if you've done the bleeding job right. She has to see your effing face in the floor'. Another woman who worked in the hospital reared eight kids in her flat near Hill Street. One of them became an accountant afterwards. It was such an achievement to get a young lad to Leaving Certificate under those dreadful circumstances. In another block of flats across the road near the labour exchange there was a family who I used to bring bananas to. My father used to say, 'There's never a banana in this house!' I also worked with Betty Heron who was a nurse and an institution in the area. She used to work mornings in St James's Hospital and come on duty in the afternoons for us. She had a great relationship with the staff in James's and used to bring Sudocrem for the sunburned children. There was nobody to show those young mothers how to raise their children properly.

The locals called the mortuary in Temple Street the 'dead house'. It was part of the lore of the inner city. Once, a young girl who I knew quite well died of a brain tumour. They had no fear of illness or death and droves of children were going up to the hospital to say their goodbyes.

I was working at Hill Street when the Dublin/Monaghan bombings went off one Friday in 1974. I was only in my early twenties and doing exams. Three explosions happened simultaneously. I never heard a bomb in my life but I put the kids in the sand pit and closed the gates. What do you do in that kind of situation but stay put? It was the first time I ever saw fathers coming to bring their children home. Betty Heron helped us to set up a kind of field hospital on the footpath. We put all the chairs out and were busy making cups of tea and putting plasters on.

That same evening I went up to Temple Street. All the hospitals had gone into red alert and Temple Street was one of the places the casualties came to. A lot of people had been injured on Parnell Street and a family of Italians were virtually wiped out. People were rushing up and down the A&E but it was very well managed. It was mostly adults who were involved in the bombs and people had gotten into a state of panic. One little child from our play centre had a very badly damaged finger – his tendons were destroyed and to make matters worse, there was a bus strike in Dublin so people couldn't get home.

In later years, I was involved with the sheltered service and adult and community education for Dublin City Council but I will always remember Hill Street and the hospital. In recent years, the area has been blighted by drugs but through the years Temple Street wasn't just a hospital – it was also a local resource; it was an early project in community development.

Rheumatic Fever Recalled

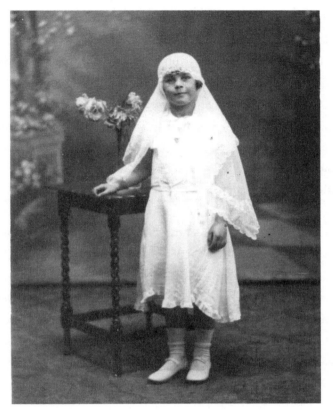

Veronica Healy pictured on the day of her First Holy Communion.
(Courtesy of Healy family)

Here, Veronica Healy (eighty-seven) recounts her experience of being a patient at Temple Street Hospital in 1936. She came from a large family and when she fell ill with rheumatic fever, it meant a three-month hospital stay – much of it spent in complete isolation from the other patients.

I came from a family of nine and was reared in Annamoe Drive in Cabra. I was the second eldest but when I was eleven years old, I was admitted to Temple Street with rheumatic fever and an enlarged heart. When I arrived, they had no bed for me so I spent my first night with my knees up in a cot. 'Don't move', they told me, 'you mustn't move'.

There was a girl used to come in because the wooden floor was varnished; she came in to polish it. She had a wooden block with a lump of lead on it and a pad under that – it was very weighty (I could tell by the way she was pushing it). 'That looks awful heavy', I said to her. 'It is', she answered, 'but I have to work'.

My mother was not allowed into the ward; when I was upstairs, there was a glass partition and I could see her through that but she couldn't get to me; underneath the glass they had cupboards so she used to open the door on her side and give in whatever she had brought; sweets and that. I could open the door on my side to receive them. I used to hate when they were taking blood. They had a punch with a needle in it and I dreaded it because it used to sting.

Because I was so poorly, I had to have complete bed rest and they meant it. I never saw the inside of a bathroom and had to be cleaned from the bed. I remember my hair being washed once. They rolled the mattress back and put the basin of water onto the bed springs.

Being admitted to Temple Street effectively finished my schooling as there was no provision for education in hospital then. The nurses used to feel sorry for me and they would bring me what they used to call 'Penny Horribles' and comics like the *Oracle* and the *Miracle*. They were love stories but I used to enjoy those. The other children were much younger than me; but then

I was moved downstairs. There was only me and a little lad in the bed opposite – he used to watch how I cracked my egg in the morning. I used to think to myself, 'Has he never seen anyone open an egg before?'

When I was ready to go home after about three months, my mother came to collect me in a push car. I was so weak, I couldn't walk. She pushed me all the way back to Cabra in that. There was no such thing as a taxi or anything. I had missed so much school and was so weak that my mother gave in to my pleading and I never went back to school afterwards.

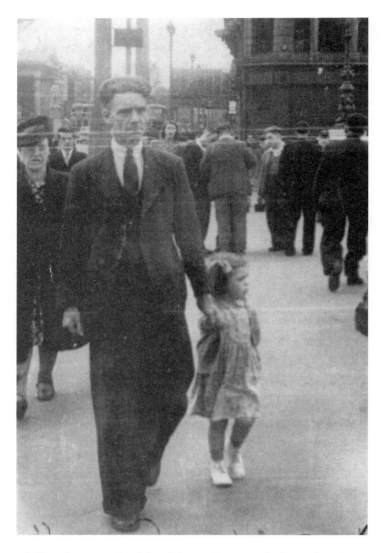

Isabelle Melia pictured with her father as they crossed O'Connell Bridge on their way to the Theatre Royal in Hawkins Street, 1949. Later that day, she was admitted to Temple Street. (Picture courtesy of Melia family)

A Case of Meningitis

Isabelle Melia, née Goulding (sixty-nine), was admitted to Temple Street shortly after the war – an experience that began with a visit to the long-since demolished Theatre Royal in Hawkins Street.

I was born on 4 November 1944 and when I was very young, we lived on Dominick Street, right across the road from Temple Buildings. My father worked as a porter for post and telegraphs and my mother was a tailoress by trade. She came from the Bolton Street area. Her father was very active in the War of Independence whereas my father's people came from around the Stoneybatter direction. We had no television and only a radio which was rented; we had plenty of time to sit around and talk and that's how you hear so many things. My mother used to tell me about what happened afterwards at Temple Street.

When I was four, we all went on a day out to the Theatre Royal in Hawkins Street. I remember Tommy Dando and how his organ used to come up out of the floor and there used to be a little screen with all the words of the song he was playing on it. A little ball used to hop along from word to word and the whole audience would be singing along – 'Keep your Sunny Side up, up, up, up'. When we got home afterwards, I felt very ill and an aunt who was home from England said, 'You better bring that child up to Temple Street; she's not well'. She thought it was unlikely that I could be so sick from just a long day out.

My parents had been to Temple Street a few years before that because I had a younger brother James who died at seven months of age; they said it was pneumonia. Today it would be classed as a cot death; he would have been between myself and my younger sister in age.

When I arrived, I was diagnosed as having a severe case of meningitis. I was immediately put into isolation. I vaguely remember being in a room and that anyone who came up to visit could only look through the window. I was treated by Dr Kavanagh during my long stay and my parents were told that my condition was very serious. I wasn't able to walk and lost the hearing in my right ear.

Then the hospital imported a new specialised drug from America for the treatment of meningitis; it was either rarely or never used before in Ireland. It saved my life. Afterwards, they sent me to Cappagh to convalesce and to learn to walk again – I was away from home for a year between everything; then they sent me then to Cork Street Fever Hospital because I caught chickenpox at Cappagh. I got measles there – both were highly contagious diseases. For a good many years after, I can remember going back to the outpatients department in Temple Street where Dr Kavanagh used to make me walk up and down to see how I was doing.

When my younger sister Mary got diphtheria, she was sent out to Cherry Orchard. Because it was contagious, you could only visit on a Sunday and I remember waiting outside the hospital gates for my mother and father. During the week, if you wanted to find out how your child was, they printed the update in the *Evening Herald*. Each patient was given a number and you could read how they were. It might read: 'unchanged' or 'progress satisfactory'.

Mothers and fathers had a lot to put up with in those days; there was a lot of tragedy but people didn't interact that much with the medical services; they had family remedies. For them a hospital was a last resort. Unfortunately I never got the hearing back in my right ear but I am happy to say that the doctors and staff at Temple Street saved my life. I will always be grateful to them for that.

A Family Tragedy

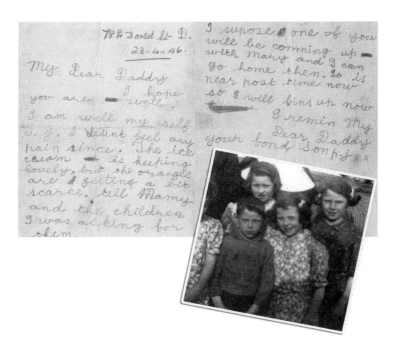

Copy of the touching letter that Philip Joseph Brady posted home on
23 April 1946, and (inset) Philip pictured with his sisters prior to his death
in 1946. (Pictures courtesy of Brady family)

*Philip Joseph Brady from Termon, County Cavan was admitted
to Temple Street Hospital in 1945 with an abdominal tumour.
Despite his illness, he had a keen intellect and between times was
still able to keep up at school. Like most children, he loved ice
cream and toffee. What follows is a moving interview with his
older sister Mary.*

We lived on a farm a quarter of a mile up a country lane in
Termon, County Cavan. P.J. was my father's first boy and after

four daughters he was understandably delighted. We all had our jobs to do on the farm. We used to make up laps of hay, turn and dry them out and drive the two horses for cutting the corn. My father made his own turf which we helped with and we were also sent out to pick potatoes. We used to milk the cows before school but P.J. was too young to do those jobs. Instead, he enjoyed climbing the ladder in the shed where the threshing machine was and getting a jaunt on the cart as all boys do. Once before school, I remember taking him to get water from the well. He slipped in but I managed to get him out in time.

When P.J. was around seven years of age, he started complaining of tummy pains. We thought it might be because he ate crab apples from the lower land about a mile away where we had a second farm. My mother and father took him to a young man in Virginia who was studying to be a doctor. He thought that the problem might be worms and referred him on for further investigation.

He was admitted to the surgical hospital in Cavan on 29 March 1945 and transferred to Temple Street Children's Hospital on 13 April where he was operated on for a bowel obstruction. The surgeons removed a tumour from his large intestine which they described as being the size of a goose egg. He was discharged from Temple Street on 25 June 1945.

P.J. was always a bright boy, even when he missed class as a result of my father taking him to fairs in Bailieborough and Ballyjamesduff, he had always been able to keep up. After his surgery, he returned to school with no problems but unfortunately his tummy pain returned and he was readmitted to Temple Street in April 1946, where the news was bad. He needed further surgery (colostomy). The pros and cons of this were discussed with our parents and, with the prospect of the cancer retuning, this surgery was decided against.

P.J. was discharged in late April into the care of his grandaunt Isabella O'Reilly, who had a boarding house and shop on Dorset Street opposite the Big Tree pub. I remember P.J. doing handstands on her couch and reciting from 'The Racing of Finn McCool' which was about a horse that won a race at Punchestown.

After that, his health got much worse. By September 1946, his legs had swelled so much that if you pressed your finger on them, they sunk right in. He was sent home to be with my parents in Cavan. I was away in boarding school in Glasnevin with my sister Agnes but we were let home at Halloween because he was very low and we helped with the night watch over him.

On the morning of 4 November 1946, we were just waiting to get the bus from Billis Bridge to Dublin when it started to rain. Dad saw that as a sign and we stayed on. Later that morning, P.J. took a turn and by two o'clock he had deteriorated further. We were all around the bed praying. It got dark early and we started to say prayers. P.J. held a blessed candle in his hands and said the night offering so clearly and with such strength of feeling that I will always remember it. 'Jesus, Mary and Joseph, assist me now, and in my last agony. Jesus, Mary and Joseph, may I breathe forth my soul in peace with you'. We were all around him. After a minute, he just turned his head to the side and died. We were all heartbroken.

On the day of the funeral, the teachers of Termon School, Miss McGlynn and Miss Harte, had the Termon school children to the house and they later marched in procession after the hearse to St Mary's Church, Clanaphilip.

A Miracle Baby

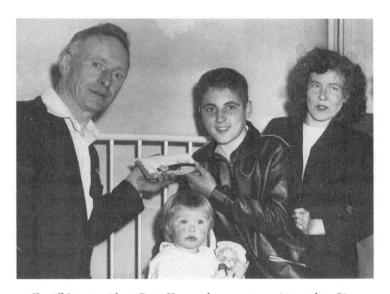

Sheriff Street resident, Peter Kavanagh presents a wrist watch to Liam Burke. The child in the cot is Baby Elizabeth (Betty) McDermott, *Irish Independent*, 5 Sept. 1960. (Picture courtesy of Liam Burke)

On 1 September 1960, Dublin's papers carried news of an astonishing lucky escape – baby Elizabeth McDermott had fallen four storeys from her flat in Phil Shanahan House, Sheriff Street, but her life was saved when she tumbled into the arms of thirteen-year-old Liam Burke. Many years later, both boy and baby were reintroduced when Liam appeared as a surprise guest at Elizabeth's twenty-fifth wedding anniversary. Here, both recount the dramatic events that led up to Elizabeth's admission to Temple Street Hospital all those years ago.

'My mother was heavily pregnant at the time', Elizabeth explains. 'She had a pot of stew on and she was washing all her paintwork in the flat. There was three of us – a four-year-old, a three-year-old and me. She said to the four-year-old, 'Keep an eye on Betty', but unbeknownst to her, I climbed up on the chair where the window was open. 'Mammy, where's Betty?' my sister said. 'I think she fell out the window'.

Taking up the story, Liam continues, 'I was coming back from Tara Street Baths along Mayor Street. At that time, they used to keep clothes lines in the flats strung from one window to the other. As I came to Phil Shanahan House, the first thing I seen was clothes falling off a line. A baby was up on the window pulling at it. I started roaring for someone to take her in. Then she fell – four storeys down. Instinctively, I put my hands out but the ground was wet and as soon as I caught her my two legs came from under me; I did a somersault and the two of us hit the ground. I jumped up and only the back of my hands was scraped. There seemed to be a bit of blood in the baby's ear. Mrs Rooney from the flats took her off me then. She ran out in the main street and stopped a car; some man gave them a lift to the hospital.

Afterwards, I came home. I just washed me hands and tidied up and had me tea; then the photographers arrived from the *Evening Herald*. They wanted to know where the boy was that was after saving the baby. She was kept in hospital for several days and I had a photograph taken there with her.

Afterwards, the local tenants got together and presented me with a gold watch; I got invited to the carnival on ice by *Tatler Press*. It was in the National Stadium and they sent a limousine down for me parents and grandparents. When we were there, a spotlight came on me and a voice announced, "There is a hero in our midst this evening." They introduced me to the crowd and then I went to the bar and got a lemonade; I had a photograph taken with the Lord Mayor, Maurice Dockerell'.

Elizabeth concludes, 'When I fell out the window, it left my father in bed for three days. He was that shook up over it. The doctors told my mother that I should have been dead before I was halfway down but I only bit my tongue. Now I have eight children and I'm a grandmother. Sure I'm still only a young one yet'.

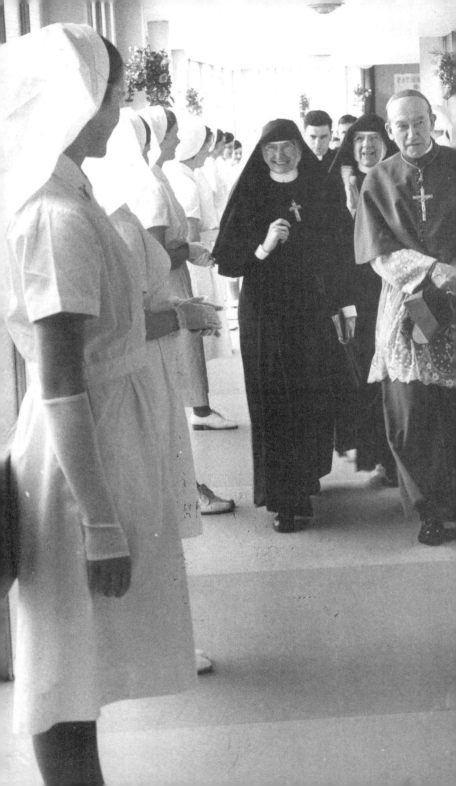

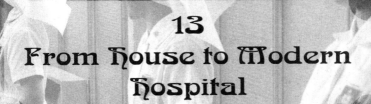

13
From House to Modern Hospital

Mother Teresa Anthony inspects new nurse graduates
on Our Lady's Corridor with Archbishop John
Charles McQuaid. The corridor joined the A&E and radiology
departments to the main hospital for the first time.
(Hospital collection)

Since its humble beginnings, Temple Street Hospital has continued to grow and expand, not just to meet the demands on its inpatient and outpatient services, but to introduce new specialties and secure its place as a teaching institution. Several key periods stand out – the 1880s when the main block was developed, the 1930s when the sweepstakes made further expansion possible and the 1970s and 1990s when Temple Street became less of a house and more a modern hospital.

In the meantime, there were other developments. At the turn of the twentieth century, a convalescent home was badly needed to care for children with tuberculosis. In 1908, Lady Martin, daughter of the famous Victorian physician, Sir Dominic Corrigan, bequeathed her lands and a large house at Cappagh, North County Dublin to the Sisters of Charity. In 1913, the Archbishop of Dublin provided them with a carriage so that patients could be transferred from Temple Street in comfort.[191] For the most part, they suffered from tubercular bone disease and treatment was carried out along the lines of heliotherapy (sunshine) and splintage. Cappagh remained in use for that purpose until 1920, when it became an orthopaedic hospital and the staff of Temple Street helped to raise funds for the project.

In 1914, a new outpatient department replaced an earlier wooden structure at Temple Street. Modelled on one of the foremost paediatric centres in Vienna, it housed a pharmacy, pathological laboratory and theatre. 'Pitch pine polished flooring will be adopted in some of the rooms', the *Irish Builder* announced. 'The glazed partition screens and principal interior doors will be mahogany and teak wood, French polished'.[192] The

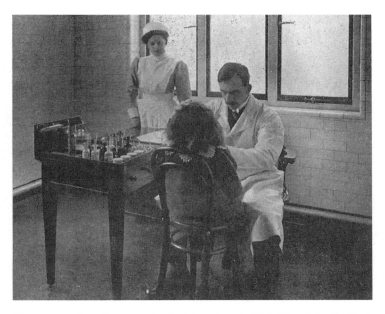

Doctor at work in the new outpatient department, 1914. (Hospital collection)

date of construction, along with the Sisters of Charity motto, *Caritas Christi Urget Nos* (the love of Christ compels us), is still clearly visible over the doorway.

The next great wave of redevelopment did not take place until the 1930s. The central hospital staircase was removed and a new ceiling installed in what is now the front hall. St. Patrick's Ward for infants was built and placed under the care of Miss Mia Rotter from Professor Moll's renowned Vienna clinic.[193] A new wing, comprising two storeys, was built at the back of No. 13. The top storey was named St. Patrick's Ward and was used for dietetic cases. It had space for sixteen cots. At its southern end was a veranda, enclosed by a large Vita glass window to allow children access to fresh air and sunshine when the weather was good. The ground floor

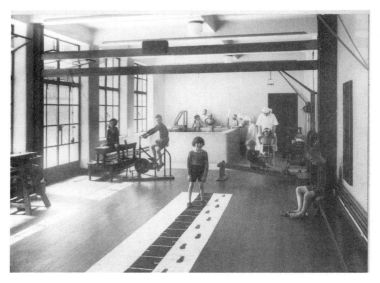

Physiotherapy department at Temple Street, c.1933. (Hospital collection)

housed a physiotherapy department with a rowing machine, exercise bike and medicinal bath.

For the first time, the hospital could begin to tackle the problem of cross-infection. Wards on all floors were divided into sections on either side of a central corridor shielded by heavy plate glass. Another room was renovated to house a new sterilising plant.

There had been an X-ray department at Temple Street since 1907, under the management of Dr Henry Mason, but it was difficult to use the equipment for anything other than breaks and fractures because patients needed to be kept immobile for long periods of time – something akin to an MRI scan today. In the 1930s, a new machine was installed. Powered by a massive basement generator, it featured an oil-cooled tube and four-valve rectification set. At a stroke, radiological exposure times were

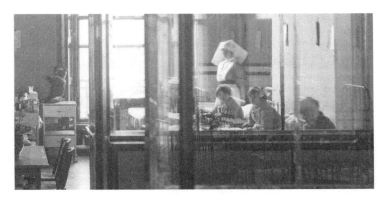

St. Agnes Ward (Surgical Flat) was divided by Vita glass for the first time during the 1930s. Note the curious children and teddy bear propped up on a bed stand. (Hospital collection)

reduced to hundredths of a second. Treatment was provided free of charge but nevertheless, exposed films were still stored in the main hospital, which was a fire hazard, and a new building was badly needed.[194] One retired staff member recalls:

We used to have to develop our own films in the dark and we used a fixer to stop them over-exposing. You had to work on developing those images in the dark and God help you if you fumbled and let a roll fall out of your hand – you would end up scrambling around for it in the dark. You got quite used to the taste of fixer on your sandwiches! Sometimes, we used to bring wet films down to the A&E department if there was something that needed to be seen in a hurry. That meant bringing the films down the long corridor – you could follow the drips! An occupational hazard was if you left a packet of films on a hot pipe because they would end up being melted. The sisters in the hospital were very industrious too. They used to collect up the used films, wipe the gelatine off them and fashion them into lamp shades and book covers.[195]

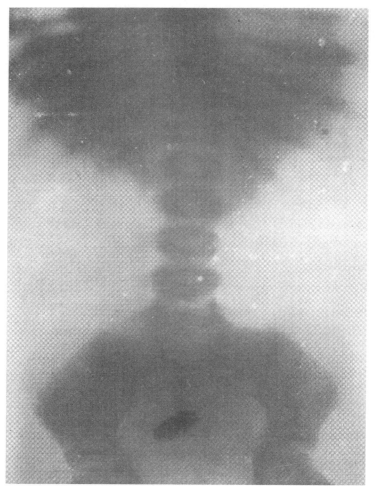

Skiagram of halfpenny in child's abdomen, taken at Temple Street in 1911.
(Hospital collection)

From House to Modern Hospital

By the end of the decade, the hospital had succeeded in making the transition from a charitable infirmary to that of a modern healthcare facility. Funding from various sources such as the hospital sweepstakes enabled the construction of other badly needed services including a milk kitchen, a new operating theatre, a plaster theatre and St. Michael's Ward.

Heating, hot water and electrical services, however, continued to lag behind such advances. During the post-war years, there was very little electrical equipment in the hospital. Nurses took a patient's pulse by applying a finger to the wrist and there were only a handful of sockets. Every day, twenty bags of coal and the same of slack were delivered to run the Cornish boiler with eight additional coal-fired boilers dotted around the hospital. But since the steam was only kept running until the laundry finished at three o'clock, fires still had to be lit every evening on the wards. Nineteen thirty-six was a particularly harsh year due to the coal strike in Dublin and the children suffered greatly when the hospital ran out of supplies – particularly those who suffered from pneumonia. Facing the prospect of having to close the hospital laundry, the sisters pleaded with the strike committee but their request for coal was refused.[196] Many years later, a pitiful note was found on the back of an old cigarette packet at the bottom of the hospital lift shaft that read something like – '1936: this was a bad year for little babies. We lost a lot of children'.

Despite such difficulties, hospital services continued to develop. In 1959, Sr Marie de Montfort, known as 'the cycling nun', started a speech therapy clinic in the old outpatients department. She was one of the first people in the country to hold a licentiate from the College of Speech Therapists (London) and her department proved to be a huge success. Nevertheless, it was

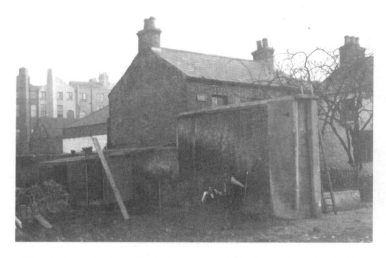

This photograph shows the bottom corner of the hospital garden looking towards Home Cottage, 11 November 1937. The large wood pile seen to the left would suggest that the sisters occasionally resorted to other types of fuel – perhaps in response to the deprivation of the previous winter. (Hospital collection)

a department that was still in its infancy, as Sr Mary Threadgold explains: 'Back then we used the general term of dyslalia for many of the conditions we encountered'. In September 1961, the *Irish Independent* reported:

> Altogether since the foundation of the Temple Street therapy department 750 children have passed through its playroom where the little patient at once begins to feel at home loses his shyness and talks for the first assessment. Tape recorders are also brought into use both for adults and children so that they may hear their own voices and learn to correct their faults. They also mark the progress that is being made.[197]

Six years later, St. Frances Clinic was opened. It was soon home to a number of complementary services such as psychiatry, psychology and audiology.

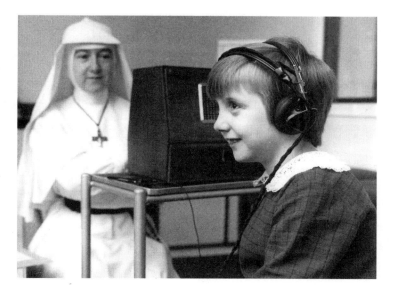

Audiology and speech and language therapy were complementary services at Temple Street and the sisters who ran the department were highly trained professionals. (Hospital collection)

During the 1960s, Mother Superior Sr Canisius O'Keeffe was instrumental in helping to link separate parts of the hospital for the first time. While looking out her office window during the depths of winter, she watched a nurse walking through the garden with a child in her arms on her way to the main hospital – a situation that resonates with other staff members. Retired nurse Teresa Collins recalls:

We had a twelve-year-old patient with hydrocephalus who died on the ward. Two of us young nurses had to carry her across to the mortuary through the garden wrapped in a sheet. We were only seventeen years old and it was a very difficult thing for us to do.[198]

Because of these difficulties, Mother Canisius commissioned a link passage called Our Lady's corridor which joined the main hospital to the casualty department. One of my uncles was involved in the job. It would cut her office in half but before it could start, the old fire grate had to come out. The hospital was paid a visit by the Georgian Society, who thought that a few love letters from Charles Stewart Parnell's time might be hidden in the chimney stack. The grate was taken out with great care and although no letters were discovered, they decided to save the mantelpiece. Unfortunately it fell on the way into the laundry and broke into bits. Around the same time, an assembly hall was also built which featured a fine Tudor-style ceiling whose blue velvet stage hangings complemented Dr John Murphy's Christmas pantomimes. During one performance, the damsel said, 'Marry me' to which a little voice piped out from the audience – 'Oh no you won't. That's my daddy!'[199]

1966 was another ground-breaking year for Temple Street. For the first time, a screening service for phenylketonuria (PKU) was established under the direction of Consultant Histopathologist, Dr Seamus Cahalane. The aim of the programme was to test newborn infants within a week of birth via a heel-prick test to discover whether or not they were deficient in an enzyme, which could cause mental retardation if left unchecked. Previously, Dr Doreen Murphy had successfully treated a PKU patient named Gerry Murray at the hospital, as Teresa Collins explains: 'She started Gerry on a phenylalanine-free diet but it wasn't very nice. It was like grey starch'.[200] The new screening service helped to ensure that treatment could be afforded to all Irish children in future. Professor Philip Mayne writes:

> Although Dr Cahalane had trained primarily as a histopathologist, he was particularly interested in developing micro-analytical methods for investigating small samples from children. It was this interest that brought him in contact with Dr Robert (Bob) Guthrie in 1961. Bob Guthrie had developed a simple microbiological method for measuring phenylalanine levels from a few drops of blood in his laboratory at the Children's Hospital at Buffalo, New York.[201]

A system of blood tests was quickly established to ensure early detection of this genetic disease in the newborn, with necessary materials for specimen-taking made available to all maternity hospitals and registered doctors in the health authority area. These were returned to Temple Street on filter paper in prepaid addressed envelopes.[202] If a child was found to test positive for PKU, he was immediately started on a low phenylalanine diet. It was a breakthrough in preventative medicine and today, the ubiquitous 'Guthrie Card' is still in use throughout Ireland.

During the same decade, the idea of building a new hospital was first proposed. In 1967, Sr Teresa Anthony wrote to the Archbishop of Dublin to outline her plans of moving further north of the city. The idea was later abandoned in favour of constructing a new hospital on the same site. 'May we have Your Grace's approval to open negotiations with our legal advisors and those of the Dublin

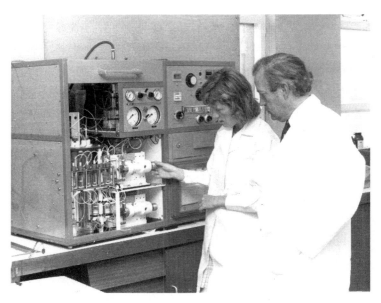

Dr Seamus Cahalane with biochemist Niamh Hynes. The machine pictured here was an early homemade amino acid analyser, produced and maintained by a German gentleman named Lockhart. (Hospital collection)

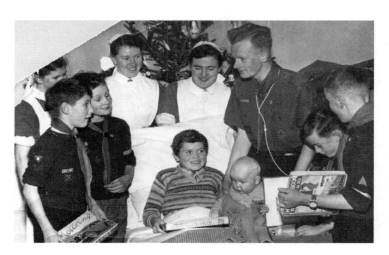

Gerry Murray, one of the first phenylketonuria patients to be treated by Dr Doreen Murphy (1955–1958). He is pictured here with nurses Mary Burke and Teresa Collins as well as with members of the Glasnevin 19th Dublin Wolf Pack, 24 December 1957. (Hospital collection)

Corporation?' Sr Anthony asked. 'They are anxious to obtain some sort of answer if we are interested and we are!'[203]

Although nothing was drawn up on paper, hospital management decided to take prudent steps with respect to any future projects at Temple Street. In 1968, a government-appointed committee on hospital services declared that there were too many small hospitals in Ireland. Its report recommended that Temple Street should be 'closely associated' with a major hospital group on the Mater site, to incorporate specialist units from Jervis Street and St. Lawrence's Hospitals.[204] The 1970 Health Act, however, did not adopt any of these recommendations. At that point, it must have become clear to the management team at Temple Street that for the time being, they would have to continue to develop services at their existing location.

Prior to the construction of a new radiology department funded by Billy Butlin and the Variety Club of Ireland in 1970, the Department of Health would only sanction foundations for a standalone building. The story goes that during a critical meeting an architect said to Butlin, 'We're wasting money putting in foundations for a single-storey building in the middle of a confined site. I want to put in foundations so as we can go up. They may be a bit superfluous at the moment but in years to come, we'll regret not having put them in'.

In response Butlin is said to have asked, 'How much will it cost to put in the foundations you want?'

When the architect told him, Butlin just took out his chequebook.

'Put in your foundations. You're the only one talking sense in this room. Now I have a plane to catch and I can't sit here listening to any more rubbish'.

On 25 August 1970, Butlin laid the foundation stone of the new X-ray unit and presented a cheque to the hospital for £3,000. Later, at a dinner held in his honour, one of the serving staff put her foot through a rotten piece of floorboard in the front parlour. 'Just keep serving and smiling', the hospital manager Lily Butler told her.[205]

The next project with which the club was involved was the construction of a new laboratory. A new amino-acid analyser took pride of place. *The Irish Times* of 27 August 1971 described the use to which this modern marvel would be put. It would be instrumental, it revealed, in 'the early detection of hereditary metabolic disease'. Other money given by the Variety Club went towards the provision of scholarships for doctors, a mobile laboratory and baby care units.

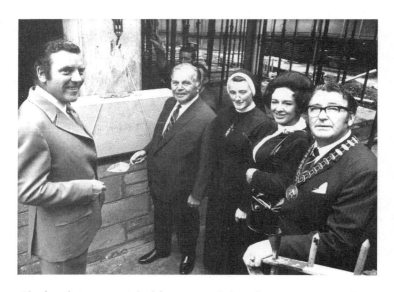

The foundation stone is laid for a new radiology department. Pictured are Mr Eamonn Andrews, OBD, Sir Billy Butlin, MBE, Mother Superior Ann Eucharia, Mrs Andrews and Lorcan Burke, chief barker of the Variety Club of Ireland, Tuesday, 25 August 1970. (Hospital collection)

From House to Modern Hospital

In 1972, the Minister for Health commissioned a local committee study group on children's hospitals which recommended that paediatric services be amalgamated into two children's hospitals in Dublin: at Crumlin and Temple Street.[206] Under the plan, Harcourt Street and St. Ultan's were to close with a new 300-bed, eight-storey hospital proposed for the Temple Street site, mirrored by similar expansion at Crumlin. The old wards at the front were to become an administration wing and a new entrance to casualty would be built at the side of George's Church. The A&E laneway which cut through the middle of the site belonged to Dublin Corporation and in order to secure possession of it, the management team struck a deal – in 1977 the Corporation granted ownership of the laneway in return for which the hospital handed over two houses on Temple Street. These were subsequently knocked down to create the lane where the IMPACT trade union building is today. A subway was built between the convent and main hospital so that the nuns did not have to go onto the street.

The project was ready to go out to tender in June 1977 when a new Fianna Fáil-led government under Jack Lynch took office. The architect rang the mother superior and said, 'The Government is gone,' to which she replied, 'We had better hold off and wait until the new cabinet is appointed'. When Charles Haughey took office as minister for health, he sent word back that, having gone through the books, his department would not be able to fund the project and the plan was shelved.

In 1984, the Department of Health announced another ambitious plan for the construction of a new paediatric hospital on the site of the old one but once again it had to be abandoned due to health service cutbacks. Nineteen eighty-seven was a particularly difficult year for Temple Street. Rory O'Hanlon's decision as minister

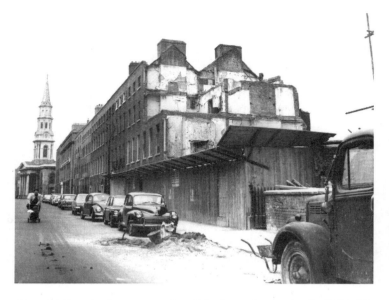

Two old Georgian houses were demolished to make way for the IMPACT lane. (Picture courtesy of Yvonne Thompson)

for health to slash the hospital budget by £1 million led to protests and staff took to the street with placards. The following year, the hospital's position was reassessed with further plans put on the table. This time, a new hospital would be built on a site adjoining the Mater Hospital. On 7 June 1989, *The Irish Times* quoted Minister O'Hanlon's promise that 'it would be a "stand alone" hospital'.[207]

In the meantime, Temple Street continued to meet the needs of sick children. The 1990s witnessed a dramatic flurry of redevelopment on a par with that of the 1930s. Some highlights included the annexation and restoration of St. George's Hall for student lectures, replacement of the old cage lift that ran through the main hospital and the conversion of St. Brigid's into a dedicated metabolic ward. The old convent on the top floor became a neurology unit and a second storey was added to the outpatient department. Towards the rear of the hospital, the old pre-fab buildings were demolished to make way for St. Ultan's Metabolic Unit and the old assembly hall – the venue for many Christmas pantomimes – made space for a new A&E department and day ward. For many, the disappearance of the hospital garden was a big loss. This author remembers the summer barbeques, the marquee tents and the music – staff reclining on the little lawns during the summer and the sweet smell of steam from the boiler house. Nevertheless, it was a small price to pay for a well cared-for child.

Nineteen ninety-eight was a landmark year for Temple Street when, amid little fanfare, trusteeship of the hospital was handed over to the Congregation of the Sisters of Mercy. For the first time in over 120 years, Temple Street was in new hands and it signalled a renewed determination to build the hospital that Irish children deserved. In 2000, plans were drawn up to construct it on the Mater site, but six years later the HSE-commissioned McKinsey & Company report revealed that according to international best practice, it ought to comprise an amalgamation of Dublin's three paediatric centres – Tallaght, Crumlin and Temple Street. A single paediatric tertiary centre was best suited to a population up to five million, ideally co-located with an adult teaching hospital (i.e. within walking distance) and preferably tri-located with a maternity facility.[208] The importance of this principle was subsequently outlined to various review groups including the Joint Task Group (2006), RKW Framework Brief (2007), KPMG review of Dublin Maternity Services (2008) and Independent Review (2011). The concept of the National Children's Hospital was born.

For the first time, complementary disciplines such as neurology and neurosurgery could work side by side and sub-specialties could be developed in many other departments. Clinical Director Dr Colm Costigan adds:

The new hospital would allow us to run specialised clinics which would be great for parents. Families could come and get everything done on the same day without their child's care being fragmented. The other thing to do is to empower the specialty groups within the city to set the model of care for that specialty around the country. There will be different models for different specialities and some of that is happening already.[209]

The Mater Children's Hospital Development group made its own submission and on 9 June 2006 a decision was made to bring the three hospitals together on the Mater site, at a cost of €650 million, in a new 445-bed centre, right beside the proposed Metro North underground station. A fifth of the money was to come from charitable and philanthropic sources, with the hospital ready to open its doors in 2016. To that end, the Sisters of Charity and Sisters of Mercy established a combined development entity and a design team was appointed.

As time dragged on, however, the economy plunged into crisis and with plans for the metro shelved, questions began to be asked in political circles as to whether the location was the correct one after all. In response, the minister for health appointed an independent review group in 2011. It confirmed that the Mater site was still the best one based on a number of criteria, which included clinical outcomes and cost. 'The creation of a world class tertiary hospital will need the commitment of everyone', Minister James Reilly said, 'including all those involved in the delivery of health services to children and in our wider society'.

On 23 February 2012, plans came to a standstill once again, however, when An Bord Pleanála refused planning permission on the basis that the new hospital would constitute an 'over-development' and that, paraphrasing concerns already raised by An Taisce, it would result in a 'dominant, visually incongruous structure and would have a profound negative impact on the appearance and visual amenity of the city skyline'.[210] Not only had a great deal of time and taxpayers' money been wasted, but the children of Ireland would have to wait even longer for their new facility.

Six Dublin teaching hospitals sent new submissions to a review group chaired by Dr Frank Dolphin, but it took time to reach a decision – partly because the area required for the new hospital was so large. 'Historically, the hospitals have combined, moved and enlarged with the dispersion of population', the report commented. 'Some have stayed central, including the Mater, maternity hospitals at Holles Street and Rotunda and Children's Hospital at Temple Street. As one of the major public perception issues relates to convenience of access, consideration must be given to the location of the hospital in relation to the child population served'.[211] Several weeks of uncertainty followed, with almost nightly news broadcasts announcing the possibility of the hospital being built in Blanchardstown, Tallaght, the Coombe as well as a number of high-profile greenfield sites owned by the National Assets Management Agency.[212] A number of landowners even offered their sites free of charge. 'It has become a war, a bidding war, between the adult hospitals', Dr Roisín Healy told the *Medical Independent*, 'and the voice of children and their parents is nowhere'.[213]

Ultimately, An Taoiseach Enda Kenny stated that Dr Dolphin's report, based on the preferred option of co-locating with an adult hospital (and ultimately a maternity facility) would be the only one used to decide the location of the new hospital and its proposal to locate the facility on a site at St. James's Hospital was approved by the Dáil.[214] At the time of writing, the plan, which allows for future expansion, incorporates two satellite A&E centres in Tallaght and Blanchardstown and the design team hopes to have secured planning approval by December 2014, with construction to begin the following spring.

In the meantime, questions continue to be asked about the services available to sick children and their families. In 2011, a joint clinical initiative was undertaken by the HSE and the Faculty of Paediatrics at the RCPI which saw the establishment of a new National Paediatrics and Neonatology Clinical Programme chaired respectively by Professor Alf Nicholson and Dr John Murphy. Both doctors hold posts at Temple Street Hospital and their stated aim is to ensure a high quality of healthcare for Irish children. According to the latest UNICEF survey, which charts the overall well-being of children in twenty-nine developed countries, Ireland currently ranks ninth and while this is by no means disastrous, much needs to be done to improve things.[215] Throughout the country, many children continue to be treated side by side with adults in emergency wards – something that Temple Street doctors fought so hard to eradicate during the late nineteenth century. Not only does the current programme aim to change such practices, it hopes to introduce an agreed approach to common conditions while at the same time working hard to ensure that all children have equitable access to care, irrespective of geographical location – the so-called 'postcode disadvantage'. On 4 March 2012, the following jointly authored letter from Drs Nicholson and Murphy appeared in *The Irish Times*:

> Sir, late last week, the one million children who live in Ireland woke up with an uncertain medical future and the inevitable prospect that their medical care will fall further behind in international terms. The best care for sick children has come into conflict with the finer points of planning. A continuation of the current overcrowded, Dickensian conditions in our paediatric hospitals is simply

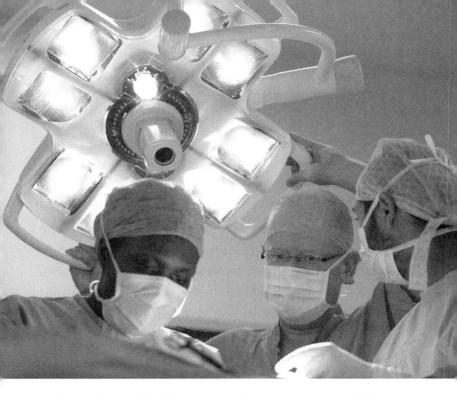

As one of Temple Street's newer specialties, neurosurgery has quickly become the busiest unit for neonates in the UK and Ireland. Depicted here are Dr Tafadzwa Mandiwanza, Mr John Caird and Mr Malinka Rambadagalla. (Picture courtesy of Ray Lohan, RCSI)

not acceptable ... a single tertiary paediatric hospital is the only solution; it should be co-located with an adult teaching hospital and adjacent to a maternity hospital – and research and education are not optional extras.[216]

The words were no different in spirit to those delivered by Dr Thomas More Madden to the Spenser Commission over one hundred years earlier – a clear demonstration that Temple Street's mission has always been a broad-minded one. With the combined expertise of Temple Street, Tallaght and Crumlin, the new paediatric hospital will reach out to every child in the nation.

Conclusion

Today, Temple Street continues to maintain an international reputation. Its Georgian rooms are home to world-class health professionals, ground-breaking national specialties and some of the most cutting-edge equipment. At the same time, the demand on its services has grown almost exponentially. In 1914, the hospital welcomed approximately 20,000 children into its newly-built outpatient department; 650 children were operated on and 1,200 were admitted.[217] At the end of 2014, as outpatients celebrates a centenary of continuous use, approximately 68,000 children will have attended clinics, 6,000 operations will have been carried out and a further 12,000 will have been admitted. On top of that, the A&E department has become one of the busiest in Europe. Temple Street, which started life caring for Dublin's children, has now become a national centre that embraces airway management, paediatric ophthalmology, craniofacial surgery, inherited metabolic disorders and national newborn screening.

At the time of writing, the hospital projects team under the guidance of Kieran Downes has built on most of the open space. Wards and offices now tower over the A&E laneway like a ziggurat. 'Construction here is very specialised', Kieran explains. 'We are working in a confined site which means that we need to plan everything carefully. Before we can start work, there are often staff who need to be rehoused. That often means fitting up temporary offices, being creative with the space we have; ensuring that disruption is kept to a minimum.'[218] In recent years, the hospital campus has begun to spread out into houses on nearby

Gardiner Row, Frederick Street and Dorset Street and many of the new facilities would not be possible without the help of public donations.

Several years of setbacks in planning the new National Paediatric Hospital have inevitably resulted in disillusionment, but hospital staff remain as committed to the children in their care as they ever were. 'You have got to divorce the actual structure from the people who work here', ENT Consultant Alec Blayney says. 'The service they provide is world standard. There is a great camaraderie and I think that's because the child is central. I wish we could bottle it because you don't find that in many other places'.[219] Ombudsman for Children, Emily Logan, who trained as a nurse in Temple Street adds:

> I think the reason why I have ended up where I am now comes from these early experiences. At the heart of the issue is social justice; getting fairness for children. Parents put their trust in us and we treated that very seriously. We felt a deep sense of responsibility towards them. I have always felt that those values were deeply embedded in the culture of Temple Street. When it comes to human rights, there are certain core values – treating people with humanity, kindness and dignity. Whether in my role as a nurse or as Ombudsman for Children, those principles are the same.[220]

Thus, as the Children's Hospital closes for the last time, the event will be tinged with some sadness. Its staff may have become attached to their old house – after all, they have spent a lot of time under

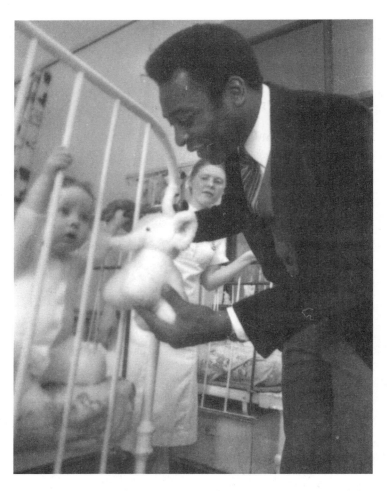

Pelé with 14-month-old Pauric McGarrigle; taken on 21 May 1979 while the footballing legend was visiting Dublin for a charity UNECEF match. In a letter to this author, he wrote 'the visit was very emotional for me'. A copy of this photograph hung in the McGarrigle family restaurant in Leitrim for many years. (Hospital collection)

its eaves as patients, employees and parents, but Temple Street has never really been about the building. In the end, it is the people and, more importantly, the children who depend on them who matter.

Bibliography

Primary Sources

Irish Military Archives (IMA)

Bureau of military history witness statements (Michael Staines), No. 284

Bureau of military history witness statements (Moira Kennedy O'Byrne), No. 1,029

Bureau of military history witness statements (Alfred Burgess), No. 1634

Bureau of Military History witness statements (Eilis, Bean Ui Chonaill – Ni Riain), No. 568

Temple Street Hospital Archive (TSA)

Temple Street Children's Hospital Annual Report, 1893

Temple Street Children's Hospital Annual Report, 1898

42nd *Annual Report of Temple Street Children's Hospital,* 1914

Temple Street Children's Hospital Annual Report, 1933

Temple Street Children's Hospital Annual Report, 1940

The Moy Mell Children's Guild – Inaugural Meeting (Dublin, 1896)

Irish Hospitals Commission Report, 1933

Irish Hospitals Commission 5th General Report, 1939-1940 and August 1941

Draft history of Buckingham Street Infirmary (Anonymous)

Documents concerning dispute between hospital consultants and Sisters of Charity (1899-1900) – one folio containing original correspondence, handwritten document chronicling the dispute as it unfolded and typescript of Dr Thomas More Madden's response to *Lancet* article 'Hospital Abuse in Dublin', 22 Feb. 1900.

Documents concerning establishment of school of domestic economy at Temple Street (1904-1915) and disbursement of funds resulting from Marcus Hughes Charity – one folio containing original correspondence, typed letters from Inspector of Industrial Schools and handwritten correspondence between Sisters of Charity and others.

Nursing Register for Temple Street Hospital (1917-1939)

Hospital account book, July 1876–January 1897

Income and expenditure book, 1912

Typewritten reports from hospital auditors and accountants (1916-1946) – several loose documents comprising précis of major projects undertaken and income and expenditure summary for year end from Kevans & Sons Auditors, Chartered Accountants and Devereux, Lynch & Co. Auditors and Accountants

Sisters of Charity Archive (SCA)

Annals of Sisters of St. Joseph's Hospital, Temple Street, 1883-1884

Annals of Sisters of St. Joseph's Hospital, Temple Street, 1899

Annals of Sisters of St. Joseph's Hospital, Temple Street, 1900-1905

Annals of Sisters of St. Joseph's Hospital, Temple Street, 1915-1921

Annals of Sisters of St. Joseph's Hospital, Temple Street, 1921-1927

Annals of Sisters of St. Joseph's Hospital Temple Street, 1941-1947

45th *Combined Annual Report of Temple Street Hospital for the Years 1915, 1916 and 1917* (419/1/2/C6)

Bibliography

National Archives of Ireland (NAI)
Property Losses (Compensation) Papers, 1916
1901 and 1911 Census of Ireland
Wills and Administrations

Diocesan Archives (DA)
Papers of Archbishop William Walsh
Papers of Archbishop John Charles McQuaid

University College Dublin Archive (UCDA)
Minute book of the Belgian Refugees' Committee, 1914-1915

Irish Architectural Archive (IAA)
William H. Byrne & Son collection (Maps and plans of Temple
   Street Hospital)

Journals, Newspapers and Periodicals
Building News and Engineering Journal, London
Dublin Quarterly Journal of Medical Science
Fingal Independent
Freeman's Journal
Irish Builder and Engineer
Irish Independent
Irish Medical Directory
Irish Monthly
The Irish Times
Journal of the Irish Medical Association
Medical Independent

Secondary Sources

Anonymous, *Our Big House and Our Tiny Bulletin* (Dublin, 1873)

Banim, Mary, *Story of the Children's Hospital Temple Street Dublin – A Sketch for Irish Children at Home and Abroad* (Dublin, 1892)

Barsoum, Noha and Charles Kleeman, 'Now and Then: The History of Parenteral Fluid Administration' in *American Journal of Nephrology*, 2002, 22, pp.284-9

Behan, Brendan, *Confessions of an Irish Rebel* (New York, 1967), p.212

Butler, Katherine, 'Catherine Cummins and her hospital: 1920-1938' in *Dublin Historical Record*, Vol. 45, No. 2 (Autumn, 1992), pp.81-90

Cameron, Charles, *A Report upon the State of Public Health in the City of Dublin for the Year 1908* (Dublin, 1909)

Campbell, John P., 'Two memorable Dublin Houses' in *Dublin Historical Record*, Vol. 2, No. 4 (Jun – Aug 1940), pp.141-155

Casey, Christine, *Dublin – The City within the Grand and Royal Canals and the Circular Road* (Yale, 2005)

Cattell, Henry W. (Ed.), *International Clinics – A Quarterly of Clinical Lectures and Especially Prepared Articles on Medicine, Neurology, Surgery, Therapeutics, Obstetrics, Psychiatrics, Pathology, Dermatology, Diseases of the Eye, Ear, Nose and Throat, and other topics of interest to students and practitioners,* Vol. 3, Eleventh series, 1901

Dock, Lavinia L., *A History of Nursing: The Evolution of Nursing Systems from the Earliest Times to the Foundation of the First English and American Training Schools for Nurses,* Vol. III (London and New York, 1912)

Bibliography

Fannin, Alfred, Adrian Warwick-Haller, Sally Warwick Haller, *Letters from Dublin, Easter 1916: Alfred Fannin's Diary of the Rising* (Dublin,1995)

Fielding, Michael, *Never Forget Them – Growing up in 1940s Dublin* (Dublin, 2010)

Fitzpatrick, David (ed.), *Ireland and the First World War* (Dublin, 1998)

Kennerk, Barry, 'Catholic Unionism and Heterodoxy in Irish Victorian Medicine: A Biography of Thomas More Madden, 1838-1902' in *Journal of Medical Biography* (Spring 2014)

Kinsella, A., 'Medical Aspects of the 1916 Rising' in *Dublin Historical Record*, Vol. 50, No. 2 (Autumn, 1997), pp.137-70

Luddy, Maria, *Women and Philanthropy in Nineteen-Century Ireland* (Cambridge, 1995)

Matthews, Ann, *Renegades – Irish Republican Women, 1900-1922* (Cork, 2010)

McPartland, Sr Magdalene (ed), *The Children's Hospital Temple Street – The Post Centenary Years – 1972-2002* (Dublin, 2002)

MacLellan Anne and Alice Mauger (eds), *Growing Pains – Childhood Illnesses in Ireland 1750-1950* (Dublin, 2013)

Meenan, F.O.C. (Ed), *The Children's Hospital Temple Street Dublin – Centenary Book* (Dublin, 1972)

Niall, Brenda, *The Riddle of Father Hackett: A Priest in Politics in Ireland and Australia* (Canberra, 2009)

O'Donnell, Barry (ed), *Irish Surgeons and Surgery in the Twentieth Century* (Dublin, 2008)

Outline of the Future Hospital System – Report of the Consultative Council on the General Hospital Services (Dublin, 1968)

Report of the Royal Commissioners appointed to Inquire into the Sewerage and Drainage of the City of Dublin and other matters connected therewith (Dublin, 1880)

Review Group on the National Children's Hospital – Report to the Minister (Dolphin Report), 7 June 2012

Russell, Matthew, 'Mrs Ellen Woodlock – an admirable Irishwoman of the last century' in *The Irish Monthly*, 36 (1908), pp. 171-6

Ryan, Patrick, *Distant Babylon* (Dublin, 2005)

United Nations Children's Fund (UNICEF), *Child Well Being in Rich Countries – A Comparative Overview* (Italy, 2013)

Internet Sources

An Bord Pleanála Inspector's Report, PL29S.PA0024 –Application under Section 37E of Planning & Development Act 2000 as amended (www.pleanala.ie), Accessed Jan. 2014

McKinsey and Company Report on Tertiary Paediatric Services in Ireland, 2006 (www.hse.ie), Accessed Jan. 2014

Interviews

Anonymous, 25 July 2013

Barry, Marie T., 20 June 2013

Blayney, Mr Alec, 29 January 2013

Bridgeman, Esther, 13 June 2012

Browning, Brian, 11 June 2013

Burnell, Tom, 17 June 2013

Cobbe, Bert, 16 May 2013

Connell, Helen, 11 June 2013

Costigan, Colm, 7 March 2013

Cunningham, Maureen, 11 June 2013

Delaney, Collette, 14 June 2013

Dempsey, Bridget (deceased), 4 July 2013

Downes, Kieran, 6 February 2014

Doyle, John, 7 January 2013

Bibliography

Dudley, Gerry, 1 March 2013

Dunne, Declan, 11 June 2013

Durney, Niall, 23 May 2012

Fahy, Sr Francis Ignatius, 8 March 2013

Foran, Michael, 2 May 2013

Funge, Annie Bernadette (née Curtis), 20 July 2012

Joly, Bríd, 12 February 2013

Keenan, Peter, 10 June 2013

Kenna, Bernie, 2 May 2013

Kennerk, Jack, 3 February 2013

Logan, Emily, 27 August 2013

McLoughlin, Eileen, 28 June 2013

Meenan, Dr Livinia, 30 April 2013

Murray, Antoinette, 9 June 2013

Nicholson, Audrey, 27 August 2012

O Ceallaigh, Ray, 27 January 2013

O'Connell, Teresa (née Collins), 16 June 2013

O'Flynn, Patrick, 2 February 2013

O'Keeffe, Rita (née Cunningham), 15 May 2013

O'Reilly, Joe, 16 May 2013

O'Sullivan, John, 23 May 2012

Randles, Catherine (Kitt), 8 February 2013

'Rashers' on www.boards.ie (Accessed September 2013)

Robertson, Lorraine (née Sheridan), 9 June 2013

Sheridan, William, 15 November 2013

Threadgold, Mary (Sr Thomas Aquinas), 2 February 2013

Endnotes

1   *Dublin Quarterly Journal of Medical Science*, 1866 and Conor Ward, 'Children's Hospital Services in Victorian Dublin: The Role of the Institution for the Diseases of Children (1822-1886)', pp.37-51 in Anne MacLellan and Alice Mauger (eds), *Growing Pains – Childhood Illnesses in Ireland 1750-1950* (Dublin, 2013).

2   Matthew Russell, 'Mrs Ellen Woodlock, an admirable Irishwoman of the last century' in *The Irish Monthly*, 36 (1908), pp. 171-6.

3   Maria Luddy, *Women and Philanthropy in Nineteen-Century Ireland* (Cambridge, 1995), p.37.

4   Maria Luddy, *Ibid.*

5   Christine Casey, *Dublin – The City within the Grand and Royal Canals and the Circular Road* (Yale, 2005).

6   John P. Campbell, 'Two memorable Dublin Houses' in *Dublin Historical Record*, Vol. 2, No. 4 (Jun – Aug 1940), pp.141-155.

7   A relative on a collateral branch of the family.

8   *Our Big House and Our Tiny Bulletin* (Dublin, 1873).

9   Rosa Mulholland and Lady Gilbert, 'Today and Yesterday in the Children's Hospital' in *Irish Monthly*, Vol. 25, No. 287 (May 1897), pp.250-55.

10 *Our Big House and Our Tiny Bulletin* (Dublin, 1873).

11 *Freeman's Journal*, 18 Nov. 1872.

12 *Our Big House and Our Tiny Bulletin* (Dublin, 1873), p.7.

13 *Freeman's Journal*, 14 Sept. 1872. In 1867, Madden had shown an interest in this subject, having edited Charles Haliday's *Statistical Inquiry into the Sanitary Condition of Kingstown*.

14 *Our Big House and Our Tiny Bulletin* (Dublin, 1873), p.4 and *Freeman's Journal*, 27 Jan. 1877.

15 'On the Datura Tatula and its Use in Asthma' in *Dublin Quarterly Journal of Medical Science* (Aug. 1863).

16 *Our Big House and Our Tiny Bulletin* (Dublin, 1873), p.4.

17 Rosa Mulholland and Lady Gilbert, 'Today and Yesterday in the Children's Hospital' in *Irish Monthly*, Vol. 25, No. 287 (May 1897), pp.250-55.

18 'Children's Visit to the Children's Hospital' in *The Irish Monthly*, Vol. 4 (1876), pp.86-88.

19 *The Irish Times*, 3 Dec. 1875.

20 Income book, July 1876 – January 1897 (Temple Street Hospital Archive, hereafter 'TSA').

21 *Freeman's Journal*, 22 Dec. 1876.

22 Of note, Atkinson was also the biographer of Mary Aikenhead – the founder of the Sisters of Charity. She also had two sisters in the order.

Endnotes

23   F.O.C. Meenan (Ed), *The Children's Hospital Temple Street Dublin – Centenary Book* (Dublin, 1972), p.5.

24   Draft history of Buckingham Street Infirmary (TSA).

25   *Freeman's Journal*, 18 Dec. 1877.

26   The hospital Income book, July 1876 – January 1897 lists a bequest of £2,500 from Stephen Simpson in July 1879 (TSA). See also: Wills and Administrations for 1878 (National Archives of Ireland, 5 Nov. 1878, p.657); Memorial of an indenture from Wilson to Margeson & others, 31 Mar. 1879 (Registry of Deeds, hereafter 'ROD', Book 16/no. 109).

27   Charles Cameron, *A Report upon the State of Public Health in the City of Dublin*, 1908 (Dublin, 1909), p.113.

28   *Report of the Royal Commissioners appointed to Inquire into the Sewerage and Drainage of the City of Dublin and other matters connected therewith* (Dublin, 1880).

29   Patrick Ryan, *Distant Babylon* (Dublin, 2005), p.31.

30   *Draft History of Buckingham Street Infirmary* (TSA).

31   *The Children's Hospital Temple Street Annual Report 1933* (Dublin, 1933), p.6.

32   Annals of St. Joseph's Hospital Temple Street 1915-1921 (Sisters of Charity Archive, hereafter 'SCA').

33   Dividing screens were originally used in Roman thermae and other public buildings but they found new and imaginative use in the designs of Italian architect Andrea Palladio. His ideas later formed the basis for late eighteenth-century Irish 'Palladianism'.

34   The library is described by William H. Byrne & Son in 1931 as the 'long parlour' (Irish Architectural Archive, Acc. 2006/142). This return was added to No. 15 after 1824. For a time, it was used as the medical boardroom. Its 'doorway' is actually a window opening with the original shutters still clearly visible.

35   Lavinia L. Dock, *A History of Nursing: The Evolution of Nursing Systems from the Earliest Times to the Foundation of the First English and American Training Schools for Nurses*, Vol. III (London and New York, 1912), p.99.

36   Efforts to save this house from a fire during the 1860s can still be seen in the blackened rafters at the top of the house.

37   *Freeman's Journal*, 23 Oct. 1879.

38   Memorial of an indenture, Bell and others to Margeson, 23 Apr. 1883 (ROD, Book 17, no. 297).

39   'Two Dublin Hospitals – St. Vincent's and St. Joseph's' in *Irish Monthly*, Vol. 12, No. 129 (Mar. 1884), pp.143-48.

40   *Building News and Engineering Journal*, Vol. 47 (London, Jul to Dec 1884) p.624. The dimensions for the ward on the first storey are given as '50ft by 20ft' whereas the two on the second storey were 'each 20ft'.

41   Annals of Sisters of St. Joseph's Hospital Temple Street 1883-1884 (SCA).

42   Mary Banim, *Story of the Children's Hospital Temple Street Dublin – A Sketch for Irish Children at Home and Abroad* (Dublin, 1892), p.15.

43   Leeches are listed in hospital expenditure books for various years (TSA).

44   *The Irish Times*, 30 Dec. 1893.

45   Barry Kennerk, 'Catholic Unionism and Heterodoxy in Irish Victorian Medicine: A Biography of Thomas More Madden, 1838-1902' in *Journal of Medical Biography* (Spring 2014).

46   W.A.L. MacGowan and Barry O'Donnell 'The Development of Surgical Training in Ireland', p.26 in Barry O'Donnell (ed), *Irish Surgeons and Surgery in the Twentieth Century* (Dublin, 2008).

47   *Dublin Quarterly Journal of Medical Science* (Vol. XXXII, Aug. and Nov. 1861).

48   Mr John P. Shanley, 'Reminiscences' in F.O.C. Meenan, *The Children's Hospital Temple Street – 1972 Centenary Book* (Dublin, 1972), pp.22-27.

49   In 1912, the hospital spent £18.9.6 on brandy and whiskey which equated to about two bottles a week (Income and expenditure book; TSA).

50   H.M. Swaine, secretary of local government board to Dr M.C. Staunton, 22 Oct. 1901 (TSA).

51   Interview with Esther Bridgeman, 13 June 2012.

52   H. McNaughton, *Clinical Teaching in Hospitals* (British Medical Association, 1877).

53   *The Irish Times*, 25 May 1949.

54   Interview with Dr Livinia Meenan, 30 Apr. 2013.

55   The 1901 census of Ireland lists sixteen nuns at Temple Street, the average age being thirty-five years old (National Archives of Ireland, hereafter 'NAI').

56   Lavinia L. Dock, *A History of Nursing – The Evolution of Nursing Systems from the Earliest Times to the Foundation of the First English and American Training Schools for Nurses*, Vol. 3 (London and New York, 1912), p.99.

57   Michael Fielding, *Never Forget Them – Growing up in 1940s Dublin* (Dublin, 2010), p.139.

58   Annals of St. Joseph's Hospital, 1921-1927 (SCA).

59   Draft history of Buckingham Street Infirmary (TSA).

60   Annals of Sisters of St. Joseph's Hospital Temple Street 1883/4 (SCA).

61   Annals of St. Joseph's Hospital Temple Street, *Ibid.*

62   Interview with Mary Threadgold (Sr. Thomas Aquinas), 2 Feb. 2013.

63   Annals of St. Joseph's Hospital, 1900-1905 (SCA).

64   Interview with Bert Cobbe, 16 May 2013.

65   Sr. Francis Regis to Archbishop McQuaid, 21 July 1964 and 29 July 1964 (Dublin Diocesan Archives, hereafter 'DDA' McQuaid papers, L68/3/1 and L68/3/2).

66   Interview with Sr. Francis Ignatius Fahy, 8 Mar. 2013.

67   Annals of St. Joseph's Hospital, 1900-1905 (SCA).

68   Mother Superior to Mr Craig, 26 Sept. 1904 (TSA).

69   Interview with Bridget Dempsey (deceased), 4 July 2013.

70   Annals of St. Joseph's Hospital, 1915-1921 (SCA).

71   *The Irish Times*, 16 Oct. 1926.

72   'Rashers' on www.boards.ie (Accessed Sept. 2013).

73   *The Moy Mell Children's Guild – Inaugural Meeting* (Dublin, 1896).

74   Luis Moreno to mother superior, November 1897 (TSA).

75   *Lancet*, 13 Jan. 1900 (Vol. 155, Issue 3985), pp.129-130.

76   Mother Superioress to Dr Michael Staunton, 2 May 1899 (TSA).

77   Mr Michael Staunton to Mother Superior, 25 May 1899 (TSA).

78   See: *Lancet*, 13 Jan. 1900 (Vol. 155, Issue 3985), pp.129-130.

79   Handwritten draft of document chronicling dispute between hospital consultants and Sisters of Charity, undated (TSA).

80   Mother Superior to Mr Michael Staunton, 3 June 1899 (TSA).

81   Handwritten draft of document chronicling dispute between hospital consultants and Sisters of Charity, undated (TSA).

82   See note written on the back of a petition to His Majesty, the King, 9 Oct. 1903 which mentions that the hospital had been closed for the months of July and August for cleaning in the wake of a scarlatina and measles outbreak (TSA).

83   Petition to Mother Superior, 5 Sept. 1899 (TSA).

84   Annals of St. Joseph's Hospital, 1899 (SCA), Dr Joseph O'Carroll to Mother Superior, 6 Nov. 1899 and Dr James B. Coleman to Mother Superior, 6 Nov. 1899 (TSA).

85   Archbishop William Walsh to Mother Superior, 8 Nov. 1899 (Walsh Papers, 28/10/14 DDA).

86   *The Lancet*, 13 January 1900 (Vol. 155, Issue 3985), pp.129-130.

87   John Walsh to Mother Superior, 30 Nov. 1899 (TSA).

88   Thomas More Madden, Pamphlet written in response to *Lancet's* 'Hospital Abuse in Dublin', 22 Feb. 1900 (TSA).

89   Annals of the Sisters of Charity, 1915-1921 (SCA).

90   *Temple Street Children's Hospital, Annual Report, 1898.*

91   Certificate from Royal University of Ireland placing St. Joseph's Hospital for Sick Children on its list of teaching institutions, 31 Mar. 1890 (TSA).

92   *Irish Independent*, 29 Dec. 1906.

93   Forty-fifth combined annual report of Temple Street Hospital for the years 1915, 1916 and 1917 (Irish Sisters of Charity Archive, hereafter 'SCA', 419/1/2/C6).

94   Margaret Downes, 'The Civilian Voluntary Aid Effort' in David Fitzpatrick (ed.), *Ireland and the First World War* (Dublin, 1998), pp.30.

95   Minute book of the Belgian Refugees' Committee, 1914-15 (UCD Archive, IE UCDA P105).

96   Peter Gatenby, 'The Meath Hospital' in *Dublin Historical Record*, Vol. 58, No. 2 (Autumn 2005), pp.122-128.

97   *42ndAnnual report of the Children's Hospital*, 1914 (TSA).

98   *Irish Independent*, 24 Dec. 1915.

99   Katherine Butler, 'Catherine Cummins and her hospital: 1920-1938' in *Dublin Historical Record*, Vol. 45, No. 2 (Autumn, 1992), pp.81-90.

100 Anthony Kinsella, 'Medical Aspects of the 1916 Rising' in *Dublin Historical Record*, Vol. 50, No. 2 (Autumn, 1997), pp.137-70.

101 Interview with Bill Cullen, 2 Aug. 2012.

102 Michael Staines account of Easter Rising (Irish Military archives, hereafter 'IMA', Bureau of military history witness statements, No. 284).

103 Moira Kennedy O'Byrne's account of Easter Rising (IMA, Bureau of military history witness statements, No.1,029).

104 *Irish Independent*, 31 January 1916.

105 Ann Matthews, *Renegades – Irish Republican Women*, 1900-1922 (Cork, 2010), p.146.

106 Anthony Kinsella, 'Medical Aspects of the 1916 Rising' in *Dublin Historical Record*, Vol. 50, No. 2 (Autumn, 1997), pp.137-170.

107 Alfred Fannin, Adrian Warwick-Haller, Sally Warwick Haller, *Letters from Dublin, Easter 1916: Alfred Fannin's Diary of the Rising* (Dublin, 1995), p.41.

108 *Irish Medical Directory, 1916* (Royal College of Physicians in Ireland Archive, hereafter 'RCPI').

109 *Henry W. Cattell, Ed. International Clinics – A Quarterly of Clinical Lectures and Especially Prepared Articles on Medicine, Neurology, Surgery, Therapeutics, Obstetrics, Psychiatrics, Pathology, Dermatology, Diseases of the Eye, Ear, Nose and Throat, and other topics of interest to students and practitioners*, Vol. 3, Eleventh series, 1901, p.264.

110 Hospital account book, 1916 (TSA).

111 *Annals of St. Joseph's Hospital, 1915-1921* (SCA).

112 W.A.L. MacGowan and Barry O'Donnell 'The Development of Surgical Training in Ireland', p.26 in Barry O'Donnell (ed), *Irish Surgeons and Surgery in the Twentieth Century* (Dublin, 2008).

113 Carol Dealey, *The Care of Wounds: A Guide for Nurses* (Birmingham, 2012), p.19.

114 *Irish Independent*, 26th Apr. 1916.

115 Property Losses (Compensation) Papers, 1916 (National Archives of Ireland, Files 163, 2288 and 4272).

116 *Annals of St. Joseph's Hospital, 1915-1921* (SCA).

117 Brenda Niall, *The Riddle of Father Hackett: A Priest in Politics in Ireland and Australia* (Canberra,2009), p.64.

118 Annals of St. Joseph's Hospital, 1916 (SCA).

119 Annals of St. Joseph's Hospital, 1916 (SCA).

120 Combined annual report for St. Joseph's Children's Hospital for the years 1915, 1916 and 1917 (SCA, 419/1/2/C6).

121 *Freeman's Journal*, 12 June 1911.

122 A report from Devereux & Lynch; auditors and accountants mentions that this was still a problem at the hospital in 1930. (TSA).

123 A.R. Walter, 'Penetrating Gunshot Wound of the Abdomen in Civilian Practice' in *British Medical Journal*, Vol. 1, No. 2980 (9 Feb. 1918), p.175.

124 Edward J. Domville, 'Gunshot Wound of Abdomen in a Boy' in *British Medical Journal*, Vol. 1, No. 2987 (30 Mar. 1918), pp.371-372.

Endnotes

125 *Sinn Fein Rebellion Handbook for Easter 1916* (Dublin, 1917), p.30.

126 Annals of Sisters of Charity, 1916 (SCA) and Kevan & Sons Auditors, Chartered Accountants, accounts for 1916 at Temple Street Hospital (TSA).

127 *Freeman's Journal*, 18 May 1916.

128 Michael McNally, *1916 – Birth of the Irish Republic* (Oxford, 2007), p.91.

129 Fifty-third detailed Annual Report of the Registrar General for Ireland containing a General Abstract of the Numbers of Marriages, Births and Deaths Registered in Ireland during the year 1916 (Dublin, 1916).

130 Spencer C. Tucker, *The European Powers in the First World War: An Encyclopaedia* (New York, 1996), p.365.

131 Forty-fifth combined annual report of Temple Street Hospital for the years 1915, 1916 and 1917 (SCA, 419/1/2/C6).

132 Ida Milne, 'Through the Eyes of a Child: 'Spanish Influenza Remembered by Survivors' in Anne MacLellan and Alice Mauger (eds), *Growing Pains – Childhood Illnesses in Ireland – 1750-1950* (Dublin, 2013), pp.159-174.

133 Annals of Sisters of Charity, 1915-1921 (SCA).

134 Annals of Sisters of St. Joseph's Hospital Temple Street 1915-1921 (SCA).

135 *Irish Independent*, 21 January 1921.

136 *The Irish Times*, 21 May 1921.

137 *Freeman's Journal*, 18 Sept. 1920.

138 Interview with Joe O'Reilly, 16 May 2013.

139 *Irish Independent*, 15 Nov. 1920 and Interview with Joe O'Reilly, *Ibid.*

140 Interview with Patrick O'Flynn, 2 Feb. 2013.

141 Katherine Butler, 'Catherine Cummins and her hospital: 1920-1938' in *Dublin Historical Record*, Vol. 45, No. 2 (Autumn, 1992), pp.81-90.

142 Statement of Eilis, Bean Ui Chonaill (Ni Riain) (IMA, Bureau of Military History witness statements, No. 568).

143 Annals of Sisters of St. Joseph's Hospital Temple Street 1915-1921 (SCA).

144 Statement of Eilis, Bean Ui Chonaill (Ni Riain), (IMA, Bureau of Military History witness statements, No. 568).

145 Statement of Alfred Burgess (IMA, Bureau of military history witness statements, No. 1634).

146 Statement of Moira Kennedy O'Byrne (IMA, Bureau of Military History witness statements, No. 1,029.)

147 Notice issued by mother superior, extracted from letter received from Hospitals Commission, 12 Oct 1940 (TSA).

148 Report from Devereux, Lynch & Co. Auditors and Accountants, 19 Mar. 1941 and 31 Dec. 1946.

149 Interview with Niall Durney, 23 May 2012.

150 *The Irish Times*, 29 Apr. 1941.

151 Interview with Gerry Dudley, 1 Mar. 2013.

152 Interview with Bridget Dempsey (deceased), 4 July 2013.

153 The nursing records for 1931 show that Ms Rotter came from Czechoslovakia. She joined on 11 May 1931 and left the hospital briefly in 1935 for a mastoid operation (TSA).

154 Irish Hospitals Commission Report, 1933 (TSA).

155 Devereux, Lynch & Co. Auditors and Accountants to Minister for Local Government, 14 Oct. 1930 (TSA).

156 *The Lancet*, Vol. 216, Issue 5595, 22 Nov. 1930 and Devereux, Lynch & Co. Auditors and Accountants to Secretary of Committee of Reference, Merrion Square, 24 Apr. 1933 (TSA).

157 The Hospitals Commission 5th General Report, 1939-1940 and August 1941 (TSA).

158 Children's Hospital Report for 1940 (TSA).

159 Interview with William Sheridan, 15 Nov. 2013.

160 Annals of Sisters of St. Joseph's Hospital Temple Street 1941-1947 (SCA).

161 Interview with Antoinette Murray, 9 June 2013.

162 Interview with Rita O'Keeffe (née Cunningham), 15 May 2013.

163 Interview with Maureen Cunningham, 11 June 2013.

164 Interview with Declan Dunne, 11 June 2013.

165 Interview with Audrey Nicholson, 27 Aug. 2012.

166 Interview with Helen Connell, 11 June. 2013.

167 Brendan Behan, *Confessions of an Irish Rebel* (New York, 1967), p.212.

168 Interview with John O'Sullivan, 23 May 2012.

169 Interview with Bernie Kenna, 2 May 2013.

170 Interview with Antoinette Murray, 6 June 2013.

171 Interview with Michael Foran, 2 May 2013.

172 Interview with Tom Burnell, 17 June 2013.

173 Interview with Alec Blayney, 29 January 2013.

174 Interview with Rita O'Keeffe (née Cunningham), 15 May 2013.

175 Interview with Lorraine Robertson (née Sheridan), 9 June 2013.

176 Interview with Eileen McLoughlin, 28 June 2013.

177 Interview with Brian Browning, 11 June 2013.

178 *The Irish Times*, 23 May 1970.

179 Temple Street nursing registers, 1917-1939 (TSA).

180 Interview with Teresa O'Connell (née Collins), 16 June 2013.

181 Interview with Collette Delaney, 14 June 2013.

182 Katherine Butler, 'Catherine Cummins and her hospital: 1920-1938' in *Dublin Historical Record*, Vol. 45, No. 2 (Autumn, 1992), pp.81-90.

183 Interview with Bríd Joly, 12 Feb. 2013.

184 *Temple Street Children's Hospital Annual Report,* 1893 (TSA).

185 *Temple Street Annual Report for 1898* (TSA).

186 F.O.C. Meenan, *The Children's Hospital Temple Street Dublin – Centenary Book, 1872-1972* (Dublin, 1973), p.31.

Endnotes

187   Temple Street Hospital Nursing Register, 1917-1939, Record 251 (TSA).

188   Interview with Teresa O'Connell (née Collins), 16 June 2013.

189   These storage tanks are now modern potable units.

190   The 'Gregory Deal' refers to an agreement made between independent politician, Tony Gregory and Fianna Fail leader, Charles Haughey in 1982. In return for Gregory's support for him as Taoiseach, Haughey agreed to significant government expenditure for the north inner city.

191   Sr. A. Joseph to Archbishop Walsh, 7 Feb. 1913 (DDA Walsh papers, Nuns, 19/12).

192   *Irish Builder and Engineer*, 2 Aug. 1913.

193   The nursing register shows that Ms Rotter joined the hospital on 11 May 1931 and that she was born in Hohenelbe in what is now the Czech Republic.

194   Report from Devereux, Lynch & Co. Auditors and Accountants, 31 Dec. 1930 (TSA).

195   Interview with anonymous, 25 July 2013.

196   *Irish Times*, 16 Apr. 1936.

197   *Irish Independent*, 26 Sept. 1961.

198   Interview with Teresa Collins (née O'Connell), 16 June 2013.

199   Interview with Alec Blayney, 29 January 2013.

200   *Ibid*.

201   *The Children's Hospital Temple Street – The Post Centenary Years- 1972-2002* (Dublin, 2002), p.104.

202   Press release on inauguration of national PKU detection service, 31 January 1966 (TSA).

203   Sr. Teresa Anthony to Archbishop John Charles McQuaid, 15 Oct. 1967 (DDA, McQuaid papers, L.68/2/1-3).

204   *Outline of the Future Hospital System – Report of the Consultative Council on the General Hospital Services* (Dublin, 1968), p.119.

205   *The Children's Hospital Temple Street – The Post Centenary Years- 1972-2002* (Dublin, 2002), p.x

206   *Journal of the Irish Medical Association*, vol. 65, issues 1-12 (1972, p.123.

207   *The Irish Times*, 7 June 1989.

208   McKinsey and Company Report on Tertiary Paediatric Services in Ireland, 2006 (www.hse.ie), accessed January 2014, p.31.

209   Interview with Dr Colm Costigan, 7 March 2013.

210   An Bord Pleanála Inspector's Report, PL29S.PA0024 –Application under Section 37E of Planning & Development Act 2000 as amended (www.pleanala.ie), Accessed January 2014, p.129.

211   *Review Group on the National Children's Hospital – Report to the Minister (Dolphin Report)*, 7 June 2012.

212   *Fingal Independent*, 24 April 2012.

213   *Medical Independent*, 17 May 2012.

214   *The Irish Times*, 20 December 2012.

215   United Nations Children's Fund (UNICEF), *Child Well Being in Rich Countries – A Comparative Overview* (Italy, 2013), p.2.

Temple Street Children's Hospital

216 *The Irish Times*, 4 March 2012.

217 Forty-second annual report of the Children's Hospital, 1914.

218 Interview with Kieran Downes, 6 Febuary 2014.

219 Interview with Alec Blayney, 29 January 2013.

220 Interview with Emily Logan, 27 August 2013.